Arteries and Veins of the Human Spinal Cord from Birth

I do not propose to learn and teach Anatomy from the Axioms of Philosophers, but from Dissections and the fabric of Nature.

WILLIAM HARVEY

Dedicated to the study of scoliosis and other deformities, injuries and diseases of the spine.

The Arteries and Veins of the Human Spinal Cord from Birth

G. F. DOMMISSE M.D., Ch.M., F.R.C.S.(Ed.)

The Department of Orthopaedics, University of Pretoria.
The Orthopaedic Hospital, The Department of Hospital Services,
Transvaal Provincial Administration, Pretoria.

CHURCHILL LIVINGSTONE
Edinburgh, London and New York 1975

CHURCHILL LIVINSTONE
Medical Division of Longman Group Limited

Distributed in the United States of America by Longman Inc., New York
and by associated companies, branches and representatives throughout
the world.

© Longman Group Limited, 1975

First published 1975

ISBN 0 443 01219 9

Library of Congress Catalog Card Number 74–82393

Foreword 1

Rational clinical diagnosis and treatment must of
necessity be based on a comprehensive knowledge of
pathological anatomy, and in this monograph the author
has given the first truly detailed account of the arteries
and veins of the normal spine and spinal cord. The
study has been meticulously conducted and recorded,
and the findings are presented in a manner which affords
much insight into those complications which are due to
an insufficient arterial supply of the various areas of the
spinal cord. It helps also in understanding why occlusion
of spinal cord arteries may be fully compensated by
the collateral circulation in some instances, and
uncompensated in others with consequent neurological
defect.

New information is supplied in respect of the complex
venous systems of the body, and of the veins of the
spine and spinal cord in their relationship to those of
neighbouring structures. In diagrammatic form the
writer constructs a panoramic view as he sees it, and in
a series of photographs taken through the lens of a
binocular surgical operating microscope, he presents
detail of important features at various levels. Further
confirmation of the thesis which he presents is to be
found in carotid angiograms on experimental animals.

The findings, all based on factual observation and
meticulously recorded, will pave the way for a clearer
concept of a number of neurological problems of
interest to the neurologist, the neurosurgeon and the
orthopaedist. For all these reasons, this inspiring
treatise becomes a valuable contribution and forms the
basis of an understanding of the minutiae of normal
cord circulation. It offers a platform from which to
launch a study of the abnormal.

February, 1974.   Professor R. LIPSCHITZ, F.R.C.S.,
Chief Neurosurgeon,
University of Witwatersrand and
the Baragwanath Hospital.

Foreword 2

The publication of *Arteries and Veins of the Human Spinal Cord from Birth* sets the seal on a detailed study of the vascular patterns of the human spinal cord carried out in the Department of Anatomy, University of Pretoria, from 1970–1973.

The aim of this study for which I had the pleasure to act as promoter, was to clarify uncertainties with regard to the rôle of the arterial supply of the spinal cord with reference to spinal surgery, and to provide useful anatomical information about the venous drainage. In this aim the author has succeeded admirably. The study further supplies the anatomist with a new meticulously worked out standardized technique of micro-dissection of the spinal cord, after filling the spinal vessels with red latex. These techniques described by the author are of a very high standard and results obtained are reliable and of great significance. In particular, findings will be meaningful in the application thereof in orthopaedic and neurosurgery.

I have no doubt that this publication will be of great value to anatomists and surgeons alike in their study of the human spinal cord in health and disease.

February, 1974.   D. P. KNOBEL, M.B.Ch.B., Ph.D.,
Professor and Head: Department
of Anatomy & Histology,
University of Pretoria.

Preface

Adamkiewicz (1881, 1882), and Kadyi (1889), wrote The Classics, in which they defined the average pattern of spinal cord circulation. With immaculate diagrams they illustrated the surface vessels (the macrocirculation), and the vessels of the substance of the cord (the microcirculation).

Suh and Alexander (1939), offered a diagrammatic representation of the computerised average version of the arteries and veins in a series of twenty-six human cadavers.

It remained however to define the variations, as well as those variants which were nevertheless within normal limits. It became necessary also to test the validity of the concept generally held, that the critical level in cord circulation was the tenth thoracic vertebra where the 'arteria radicularis anterior magna', the artery of Adamkiewicz, was often found.

To these ends, an intensive microdissection study was instituted in which the vessels of the cord and surrounding structures were exposed in forty-two cadavers.

In an additional small series, microangiograms enabled an 'instant' view of the full extent of the cord *in situ*.

In the course of a period of nearly five years the author completed the manuscript and became indebted to a number of people and institutions. The Medical Research Council of South Africa in collaboration with the University of Pretoria provided a grant in aid. The National Council for the Care of Cripples in South Africa committed itself to a subsidy which in the event was not required but was none the less appreciated.

The Dean of the Faculty of Medicine at the University of Pretoria, Professor H. W. Snyman and the Director of Hospital Services in the Transvaal Administration, Dr H. A. Grové offered the weight of their support in their personal and official capacities, and the successive heads of the Department of Orthopaedics in Pretoria, Professor G. T. du Toit and Professor I. S. de Wet were towers of strength.

In the Department of Anatomy, Professor Tobie Muller and her successor Professor D. P. Knobel placed their services at my disposal, and made the project possible.

The success of the technique of vascular injection in obtaining total filling of the arterial and venous channels, and of the photographic recording of nearly all of them was in large measure due to the persistence and perseverance of the principal technician Mr H. Brüne and staff, and of Miss H. Coetzee, M.Sc., and Mrs T. Teuben.

At the Poliomyelitis Research Institute in Edenvale, Dr Winter and staff provided the facilities for the animal experimentation, of immeasurable value in developing the technique of study.

At the surgical Department of the Veterinary Institute at Onderstepoort. Professor C. F. B. Hofmeyr and Staff enabled the continuing animal experimentation, while Professor de Boom of the Department of Anatomy was at all times available for consultation.

The Louw van Wyk Orthopaedic Trust Fund placed on loan a binocular surgical microscope.

The Superintendent of the H. F. Verwoerd Hospital in Pretoria, Dr W. J. Kenny and his successor Dr E. van Wyngaardt offered their encouragement. Hennie's Secretarial Services and later Miss H. Breedt of the Orthopaedic Department did the typing.

To these and many others I am deeply grateful.

To my wife and our family, my thanks and appreciation of sacrifices gladly made, and of unfailing understanding and patience.

There was one other factor, so well expressed by Kendall:* 'The research worker may carry on his investigations in the quiet seclusion of a laboratory, quite isolated from the busy importance of world affairs. . . . But there is an intangible and sometimes unrecognized presence which is always very near. This may be personified in the patient who comes for relief but who will not get well; in the parent who brings his child only to learn there is no help. The presence of these unseen spirits is always realized in a research laboratory, and it is for them that the investigator may well be patient and persistent.'

February, 1974.   G. F. DOMMISSE,
                    Pretoria, South Africa.

*E. C. Kendall, Nobel Laureate, 1950. In *Mayo Clinic Proceedings*, Volume 48, number 10, page 738. Historical vignette by Ruth J. Mann, History of Medicine Librarian.

Contents

1. Introduction

During the past hundred years the blood supply of the
human spinal cord has been extensively investigated and
reported, and the reports have necessarily dealt
separately with the two aspects of the subject which are:
  1. The microcirculation, which includes the capillaries
     only.
  2. The macrocirculation which includes the vessels
     from those of the seventh order to those of the
     third.
They are respectively the segmental vertebral branches
which arise from the posterior aspect of the aorta, and
the arterioles and venules which have a diameter of
16 to 32 micrometers, as defined by Alexander and
Putnam (1938).

The microcirculation has been consistently reported by
numerous workers, and recently again by Turnbull
(1971), who recorded the regional differences in the cord
as determined by micro-angiograms in a series of human
cadavers.

Not so the macrocirculation, where reports vary as the
techniques of study. Today, the details of spinal cord
circulation remain controversial. Controversies in respect
of the cerebral circulation were in large measure resolved
by Stephens and Stillwell (1969), whose monograph
entitled *Arteries and Veins of the Human Brain,*
constitutes a standard reference. In the introduction they
state: 'Early studies of the cerebral arteries concerned
only the main vessels. . . . The details of smaller
branches . . . were neglected. A few studies have been
done that concern the distribution of all or part of a
major artery. Other reports describe the arterial supply
to a specific area of the brain. Although these have
produced much useful information, nevertheless, the
details of the intracerebral arteries and their relations to
each other necessarily remain hazy. Differences in
injection techniques, the problems of collateral channels
modifying the distribution of a separately injected
artery, the distortion of the injected vessel by the
procedure, . . . and the different points of injection and
ligation have led to conflicting results. Moreover, the
lack of dependable technique to visualise the arteries
from origin to termination, in detail and without
distortion, has limited anatomical accuracy.'

The present study represents an attempt to fill the

1

need in respect of the spinal cord. A technique of study has been developed in our laboratories at the Department of Anatomy, University of Pretoria, for the selective filling of the vessels of the entire cadaver (Dommisse, 1972a). When it is desired to exclude the pre-capillaries and the capillaries, then a preparation of latex is used. When the capillaries are to be included in the study, then micropaque suspended in gelatine is injected and the same technique is employed (Fig. 1.1).

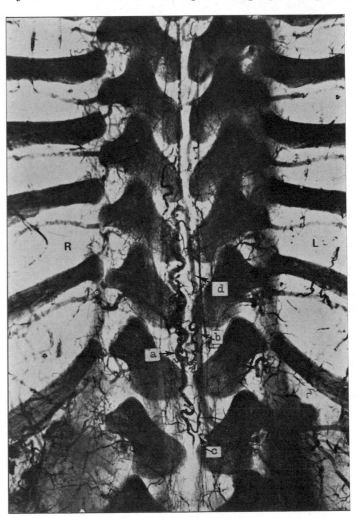

Fig. 1.1 Microangiogram of neonatal cadaver, showing relationship of arteries of supply to the spinal cord and surrounding structures.

In the first series, a detailed microdissection of the vessels down to the third order was carried out. The positive identification of small arteries and of arterioles, also of small veins and of venules was achieved in every instance of doubt, by the direct procedure of exposure of the vessel in question, from terminal extremity back to the point of origin. The fact that the cord was retained *in situ* during the dissections made the technique possible, and was responsible for removing doubt.

In a subsequent series, the technique was altered and the capillaries were filled with radio-opaque material for the purpose of angiographic studies.

By providing a photographic reproduction of the vessels at all levels in 42 cadavers, representing age groups from neonatal to pre-senile, the need for art work and an artist's impression has been eliminated. Schematic representations have been used only where needed to present the picture as a whole. Detail in all instances has been provided by through-the-lens photographs taken at magnifications of six, ten or sixteen times. Greater magnifications were used occasionally to facilitate dissections at arteriolar level.

The literature has been extensively reviewed and a great variability of report has been exposed. Suh and Alexander (1939) commented to the same effect. The causes of the variability have been sought, and have been narrowed down to four main channels:

1. The use of techniques of vascular filling which are confined to specific regions of the spinal cord rather than the whole.
2. The study of the cord after removing it from the cadaver, instead of retaining it *in situ*.
3. Reliance upon angiographic studies which although expedient, are liable to misinterpretation. Over-lapping shadows cannot be traced from origin to termination, and arterial channels cannot be positively differentiated from veins. Inadequate filling of vessels adds to the difficulties of interpretation.
4. Most important, the infinite variability of the human pattern. Variations of pattern rather than unreliability of the observers have accounted for many of the apparent anomalies. Reports which appear incompatible may nevertheless be accurate, and reflect the variability of the subject rather than the fallibility of the student.

In all cadavers in the series, the entire circulation was filled with an injection material administered by a closed pressure system. The technique of administration is described below.

AIMS AND OBJECTS
To provide an atlas and work of reference to the macrocirculation of the spinal cord. To this end, attention was paid to the following aspects:
1. The principles of cord cirulation, as opposed to the variable patterns, both arterial and venous.
2. The details of the vascular system of the cord in the varying age groups from the neonate to the pre-senile adult.
3. The possible presence of a 'critical vascular zone' of the cord in which the neural tissues are vulnerable to those factors which threaten the integrity of the circulation.
4. The factor(s) which provide that reserve or 'elasticity' of arterial supply of the cord, which accounts for the well-recognised, relative immunity of the cervical cord and the lumbar cord to injuries involving not only the skeletal structures, but also the blood vessels in the area. It seemed important to do so, more particularly in the light of the statement of Feeney and Watterson (1946) who declared:

'There exists a very close relationship between the metabolic requirements of the nervous tissue and the final distribution of intraneural vessels in the adult, a relationship which functions in such a way as to provide the nervous system with a blood supply just adequate for its minimal needs.' Woollam and Millen (1958) add this corollary:

'To put it in somewhat crude evolutionary terms, man has just as much nervous system as he can supply with oxygen and no more.'

Quadriplegia or paraplegia has developed as an unforeseen complication during the surgical management of cervical disc degeneration, scoliosis and other lesions.

On the other hand, Dwyer (1972), and Hall (1973), have reported the ligation of ten or more of the 'intercostal' and 'lumbar' arteries in the course of anterior exposure of the spine, without neurological deficit.

Indeed, these are some of the controversial factors which continue to perplex the clinician and the surgeon, and which justify yet a further study of the subject in depth.

2. Terminology and Techniques of Study

There is a lack of uniformity as well as clarity in the terms applied to the blood vessels relating to the spinal cord, and an example is the term 'the anterior spinal artery', which refers both to the great anterior median longitudinal trunk of the spinal cord, and the small paired branches of the vertebral arteries which join the latter at its proximal extremity. There are other anomalous terms such as the 'intercostal arteries' and the 'vertebral venous plexuses'.

In this monograph, the terms used and their connotations are described:

The anterior spinal artery (Fig. 2.1; Plate 1)
A small branch of the vertebral artery, which arises immediately caudal to the basilar artery. It is usually duplicated and it proceeds distally to unite with its fellow at between C1 and C6 segmental levels. The pair give rise to a single arterial channel which is placed over the anterior median sulcus, and which constitutes the main anterior vessel of the cord, referred to here as:

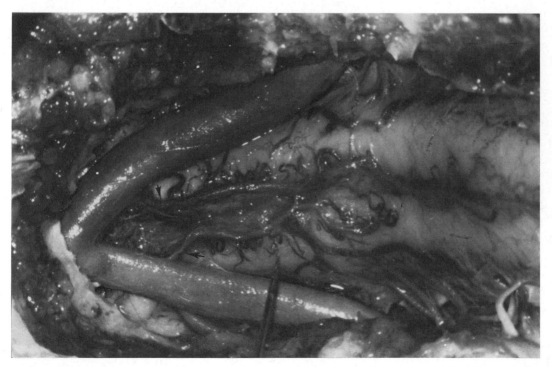

Fig. 2.1 The vertebral arteries, the anterior spinal arteries, and the anterior longitudinal arterial trunk of the spinal cord.

The anterior median longitudinal arterial trunk of the spinal cord (Fig. 2.2, Figs. 3.1–3.12; Plate 2)
The continuous compounded arterial trunk which extends from the region of the olivary nucleus of the medulla oblongata to the conus medullaris. It is placed over the anterior median sulcus. It is frequently and incorrectly termed the *anterior spinal artery*.

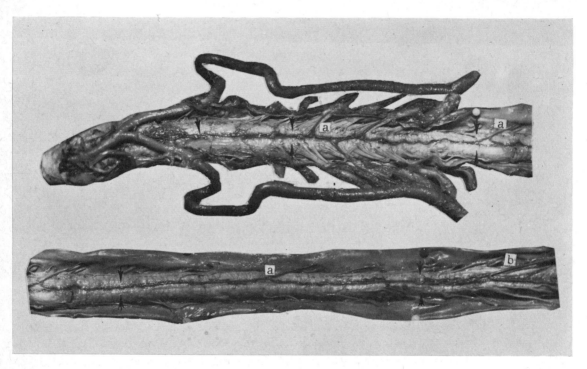

Fig. 2.2   The anterior longitudinal arterial trunk in a cord excised from the cadaver.

The posterior spinal artery (Fig. 2.3; Plate 3)
That branch of the posterior inferior cerebellar artery, or of the vertebral artery, which like its anterior counterpart is duplicated and which proceeds distally as:
The postero-lateral longitudinal arterial trunk of the spinal cord (Fig. 2.4, Figs. 3.13–3.14; Plate 4).
A continuous, compounded, ramifying vessel which extends from the medulla oblongata to the conus medullaris, and which weaves in and out among the posterior nerve rootlets. It is duplicated on the opposite side.

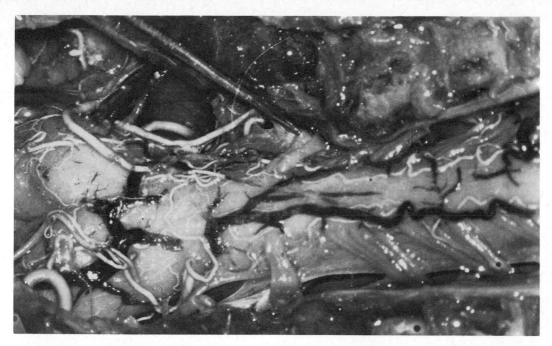

Fig. 2.3 The posterior inferior cerebellar arteries, the posterior spinal arteries and the postero-lateral longitudinal arterial trunks of the cord, which are small (white) tortuous vessels partially obscured by the posterior nerve rootlets. The (dark) tortuous midline structure is the venous channel.

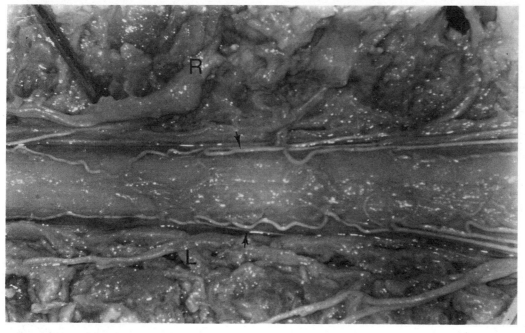

Fig. 2.4 The postero-lateral arterial trunks of the cord, clearly displayed by division and retraction of the posterior nerve rootlets. Medullary feeders are seen at T8 on right and at T7, T8 and T9 levels on left side.

The medullary feeder arteries (Figs. 3.1–3.14)
The collateral arteries of supply of the 3 longitudinal
trunks of the cord, occurring at variable levels in varying
numbers.
The radicular arteries (Plate 5)
The nutrient vessels of the nerve roots, which occur at
every level on left and right sides. They arise either
peripherally, or centrally from the longitudinal arterial
trunks of the cord. They are to be distinguished from
medullary feeders with which they may enjoy a common
origin from the segmental artery at that level.
The segmental arteries of the vertebral column (Plates 6, 9)
There is a pair of arteries at every segmental level, for
the supply of extra-vertebral, skeletal and intraspinal
structures. In the neck, they arise mainly from branches
of the subclavian artery and are duplicated at several
levels.

In the thoracic and lumbar regions they arise from
the posterior aspect of the aorta and are generally
referred to as the 'intercostal' and 'lumbar' arteries.

They will be referred to here as the thoracic and lumbar
aortic segmental arteries of the vertebral column or
simply, the 'segmental arteries'. The intercostal and
lumbar vessels are their terminal, posterior branches.
The longitudinal venous trunks of the cord (Fig. 9.2)
The anterior and posterior venous channels (Plates
20–24) which are the counterparts of the longitudinal
arterial trunks. Anteriorly there is a single trunk
which is placed over the anterior median sulcus deep
to the arterial trunk (Fig. 2.1), and into it drain the
central perforating and the pial perforating veins, also
numerous radicular venules at every segment. At the
cervical and lumbar enlargements it is often seen as a
complex system of venous channels, which are abundant
and may resemble arterio-venous malformations.
Posteriorly, a single midline trunk may be replaced in
whole or in part by duplicated or ramifying vessels
which are likewise abundant at the cervical and the
lumbar enlargements of the cord (Fig. 9.4; Plates 20–24).

The longitudinal venous trunks of the cord drain into
the inner, central portion of the plexus of Batson, that
portion described below under the sub-title 'the extra-
dural vertebral venous plexus'.

The medullary veins of the cord (Plates 20–24)
The counterparts of the medullary feeder arteries. They
accompany the nerve roots in their exit from the dural
sac, at levels which are usually not related to the
medullary feeder arteries.

They are largest and most constant at the cervical and
lumbar enlargements (Figs. 4.2, 9.4; Plates 20–24).

The extradural vertebral venous plexus (Fig. 9.6; Plates
25–27)
That portion of the plexus of Batson which occupies the
extra-dural space of the spinal canal and extends from
basi-occiput to coccyx.

It is illustrated in the thoracic and lumbar regions. It is
of interest to note that it resembles closely the 'internal
ventral vertebral venous plexus' of the domestic pig, as
described by Wissdorf (1970).

Batson (1942) described it as 'characteristically an
embryonic plexiform network of vessels'—a large venous
lake or reservoir. 'These vertebral veins have many and
rich communications with the veins in the spinal canal,
the veins around the spinal column and those within
the bones of the column' (Batson, 1940).

The vertebral venous plexus (Plates 25, 28)
This term is used in the literature to denote the several
components of the plexus of Batson and has become a
sort of generic term, lacking definition.

In this thesis the term is used in a specific sense, to
denote the plexus of veins which surrounds the vertebral
artery within the transverse foramen, and which
communicates with the cervical portion of the extra-
dural plexus at every segmental level. It communicates
also with the veins of the neck, both deep and superficial.
Proximally, it participates in the great confluence of
venous sinuses (see below), which has hitherto not been
fully described.

The great confluence of venous sinuses (Plate 25)
The participants in the great confluence of venous
sinuses at the base of the skull include:

    Those emerging from the cranial cavity.
    The deep veins of the neck.
    The superficial veins of the head and neck.
    The veins of the skull and the vertebral skeleton.

Other vessels which participate in the great confluence,
are a group of posterior veins from the neck muscles,
skin and integument, which have been described
elsewhere (Trevor Jones, 1966).

TECHNIQUES OF STUDY

Five techniques have been employed in order to cover the various aspects of the study (Dommisse, 1974). The principal method has consisted of the detailed micro-dissection of the vessels of forty two human cadavers. There were thirty neonates, one infant, four adolescent and seven adult cadavers in the series. Additional methods included:

1. Angiographic studies of the circulation of the cord in six cadavers of human neonates.
2. Carotid angiographic studies of the venous drainage of the brain in six baboons *in vivo*, using adult specimens of the species *Papio ursinus*.
3. The radiological assessment of the width of the spinal canal in fifty healthy individuals, whose ages ranged from eighteen months to sixty eight years.
4. The physical measurement of the diameters of the spinal canal in the thoracic and lumbar vertebrae in six macerated, adult human skeletons.

TECHNIQUE 1

THE MICRODISSECTION STUDY OF 42 HUMAN CADAVERS

The entire circulatory system, excluding only the pre-capillaries and the capillary beds, was filled with a preparation of latex, coloured red. The injection material was introduced through a cannula tied into the femoral artery, under a closed system and at pressures of from 34.7–137.90 kPa (5–20 psi). When a pressure of 137.90 kPa was recorded in the pump, then the intra-arterial pressure at the point of delivery was the equivalent of 1034 mm Hg.

In each instance 2–5 ml of a dilute solution of ammonia preceded the injection and produced an alkaline medium for the easy flow of the latex emulsion. No provision was made for the escape of blood, which was driven into the capillary spaces and the veins. In some instances the veins failed to fill with latex and fortuitously retained their content of dark blood. They presented as dark, brown channels which provided a sharp photographic contrast with the red of the latex-filled arteries.

The injection material was allowed to penetrate the vascular tree for periods of from five to fifteen minutes and it was noticed that while there was a rapid flow from the delivery bottle to the cadaver during the first two or three minutes, there was a much slower flow for the remaining period of the infiltration. It came to be important to observe closely the flow until it came to a gradual halt, for it was during the slow phase that successful filling of the smaller vessels was achieved. A sudden fall of pressure in the delivery system indicated the rupture of a major vessel and leakage into the tissues. In these cases, the infiltrations were immediately discontinued.

The cadaver was then embalmed. The body cavities were filled and the limbs were infiltrated as far as possible with a standard embalming fluid consisting of:

White industrial methylated spirit, 45 per cent;
Glycerine, 35 per cent;
Liquefied phenol, (85 per cent in water). 15 per cent;
Formalin, 5 per cent;
Thymol (Fungicide) approximately 0.5 per cent.

The cadavers were preserved in a half strength solution of embalming fluid for a period of two to three weeks before the dissections were commenced.

All dissections were conducted with the aid of a binocular surgical microscope of standard type, and at magnifications which proved optimal at ten and at sixteen times.

The spinal cord was retained *in situ*, while the bony skeleton was removed in sufficient amount to ensure adequate exposure yet to maintain the stability of the spine. In six cadavers the stability was sacrificed in order that both the anterior and the posterior systems of arterial supply could be observed. In these instances, stability was provided by means of external support.

Photographic reproductions were made at all levels of the cord, and included the collateral channels of the vertebral column and adjacent structures.

The vessels surrounding the spine and spinal cord were examined and recorded in detail, and the presence of arterio-arterial anastomoses noted.

The filling of veins in addition to arteries was observed in all well-injected specimens. This retrograde spread from arteries to veins has been noted also by other workers (Suh and Alexander, 1939), after arterial infusions only. It takes place through the normal arterio-venous communications of the body which have been observed in this series in the trabecular spaces of the vertebrae and the skull, and in other reports in the juxta-cortical glomeruli of the kidneys (Trueta *et al.*, 1947), in the endometrium of the uterus (Schlegel, 1945) and in the parenchyma of the lungs.

TECHNIQUE 2
THE ANGIOGRAPHIC STUDY OF SIX HUMAN NEONATAL CADAVERS

The preparation of the cadavers was the same as in the series reported above, but the injection material used was micropaque 25 per cent, alone and in combination with gelatine, 10 per cent. 20–30 ml of the former was injected by a sufficient amount of the latter (100–130 ml), to achieve maximal filling.

Special attention was paid to the temperature of the cadaver, the injection material and the apparatus. The latter, which included the delivery tubes and the gelatine mixture were heated to 60°C, and the cadavers were slowly warmed to a little more than body temperature.

Embalming was carried out as described above, and the injection material allowed to gel and fix for not less than fourteen days. The radiographic examinations were progressively carried out after the removal of as much of the bony skeleton as was necessary. Medical X-Ray film, no screen type, very fine grain for mammography, was used for the purpose.

TECHNIQUE 3
CAROTID ANGIOGRAPHY IN EXPERIMENTAL ANIMALS

Six baboons of the species *Papio ursinus* were used.

The animals were anaesthetised and the trachea intubated. The common carotid artery was exposed and cannulated with a tube or a needle of maximal bore in order to ensure rapid delivery of the injection material.

The arterial phase of the cerebral angiogram was observed after the rapid administration of 20 ml of 76 per cent Urografin. The time interval between the arterial and the venous phase was recorded in each instance by means of radiographic screening. Rapid repeat films to secure standard exposures of both the arterial and the venous phases were recorded.

Using the same animal, the internal jugular veins on the two sides were then exposed and ligated. The injection of contrast medium was repeated, and further serial films were taken.

Using the same animals again, the external jugular veins on both sides were exposed and ligated, and the angiograms were repeated.

Two of the animals were observed for a period of eighteen days following the procedure, and there were no ill effects which could be ascribed to the multicentric, jugular venous ligation. Carotid angiograms were repeated, using the common carotid artery on the other side. The arterial and the venous phases of the angiograms were again recorded.

The animals were then destroyed, and the cadavers were prepared and preserved for microdissection study.

TECHNIQUE 4
RADIOGRAPHY IN THE MEASUREMENT OF THE SPINAL CANAL IN 50 HEALTHY PERSONS

Radiographs were taken under standard conditions of the erect spinal column of 50 healthy people whose ages varied from eighteen months to sixty eight years.

The interpeduncular spaces of the thoracic, the lumbar and the first sacral vertebrae were measured and recorded. This was used as a measure of the relative width of the spinal canal at each of the several vertebral segments.

TECHNIQUE 5
THE MEASUREMENT OF THE SPINAL CANAL IN SIX CADAVERS
The antero-posterior and the lateral diameters of the
spinal canal in the thoracic and lumbar vertebrae of six
adult human skeletons were measured with a Vernier
scale and recorded. The relative dimensions at the
different vertebral levels were compared with those of
Technique 4.

SUMMARY OF TECHNICAL METHODS
The present study represents an effort to define those
features of spinal cord circulation which may be
accepted as within normal limits and to this end a
method of study developed in our laboratories at the
Department of Anatomy of the University of Pretoria,
has enabled the selective filling of the vessels of the
entire cadaver. When it was desired to exclude the
pre-capillaries and the capillaries, then a preparation of
neoprene latex was used which penetrated to vessels
having a lumen of 20–32 μm only. When the capillaries
were to be included in the study, then micropaque solution.
suspended in gelatine, was administered in the same
manner. When the filling of the arterial vessels was
satisfactory, then in many instances there was
coincident filling of the venous channels. This
phenomenon was recorded also by Suh and Alexander
(1339) and others, and is accounted for on the basis of
reverse filling via the normal anteriovenous shunts which
are located in the vertebral bodies and between the
diploic layers of the skull (Dommisse, 1972A), in the
juxta-cortical renal glomeruli (Trueta *et al.,* 1947) in the
endometrium of the uterus (Schlegel, 1945), and in the
pulmonary circulation.
   Use was made of experimental animals for the study
of a particular aspect of the venous plexus of Batson
(Batson, 1940).

3. The Arteries and Arterioles of the Human Spinal Cord

THE PRINCIPLES AND THE PATTERNS OF ARTERIAL SUPPLY

GENERAL OBSERVATIONS

Spinal cord circulation is easier to understand when seen as part of the whole (Fig. 1.1). To this end the entire circulatory system has been filled and the cord vessels have been studied *in situ*. A common source, the segmental vertebral arteries, has been shown to supply not only the spinal medulla, but also the surrounding structures such as the spinal membranes. the nerve roots, the bony skeleton, the paravertebral muscles, the autonomic nerve trunks and ganglia, and regional structures.

The spinal cord is more abundantly supplied with blood vessels at the neonatal stage than at any other stage in the growth and development of the individual. Weight for weight, it enjoys a six times advantage over the adult cord, in response to the metabolic demands of the growing neural organ.

The size of the anterior arterial vessels has been recorded in thirty six cadavers, and of the posterior vessels in eighteen cadavers. The detailed patterns of 36 of the anterior study group are illustrated (Figs. 3.1–3.12), and of six of the posterior group (Figs. 3.13–3.14). It will be observed that in some cases the adult vessels are no larger than those of the neonate, while in others they are twice as large. In most cases they are only about half as large again, and in these cases the volume of the blood flow (which is proportional to the diameter of the vessel), is only twice as great in the adult as in the neonate. This was a surprising yet consistent finding in the series, and was in sharp contrast with the disproportion in weight and volume of the cord in the respective age groups. The adult cord weighs about thirteen times as much as the neonatal, and displaces about thirteen times the volume. (*See* Chapter 7.) These figures serve to emphasise the great metabolic demands of the neural tissues during the process of growth and development, and by contrast to focus attention upon the statement of Feeney and Watterson (1946) that 'the nervous system (is provided) with a blood supply just adequate for its minimal needs'.

The variability of the arterial pattern in individual

15

cadavers has proved a dominant feature and in this series no two cases were alike. Furthermore, there was only one out of 36 cadavers in which the pattern bore a reasonably close resemblance to the computerised 'average version' of the pattern of the anterior medullary feeders offered by Suh and Alexander (1939), in a report on 26 cadavers. In their average version, the artery of Adamkiewicz (Kadyi, 1889) occurred at T10 level on the left side, and there were additional feeders at C3, T3 and L2 levels on the left side, and at C5, T1, T5 and L5 levels on the right side. In the present series, the artery of Adamkiewicz was at levels varying from T7 to L4, and on the right side in 17 per cent of cadavers (*See* Chapter 6). In the present series, the spacing of the feeders has conformed to the principle of maximal concentration at the cervical and the lumbar enlargements but with great variation in number and precise segmental levels.

The writer is, therefore, opposed to the concept of an average version of the feeder pattern, lest it lull the spinal surgeon into a sense of false security which particular care to conserve the tenth segmental artery on the left side may bring. The frequency of anterior and of posterior feeders at every level is indicated in Figures 3.15, 3.16. They may be found at any level in the individual patient and they may be crucial wherever they are found.

It follows as a corollary that angiography and, if possible, selective angiography, is indicated when it is necessary to determine the pattern in the individual patient. Djindjian *et al.* (1970), Keim and Hilal (1971) and Di Chiro *et al.* (1970), have recorded their techniques and results. Clearly, the procedure is for the esoteric and can be undertaken only by those skilled in this specialised field. Equally clearly, the fear of complications in those patients in whom vascular insufficiency is suspected will act as a deterrent.

The indications for selective angiography are equivocal, and while the need to determine individual patterns in the thoracic and lumbar regions will occasionally arise, the principles, which are constant and which are applicable in all instances, are of fundamental practical value.

THE PRINCIPLES AND THE PATTERNS

There is a basic simplicity underlying the complex patterns of the vessels of the cord, because the patterns conform to a set of rules which are referred to here as 'the principles'. The principles, which are defined below, are those features of cord supply which in this study, and in a review of the literature, have proved constant.

1: The segmental arteries of the vertebral column supply the medullary feeder arteries

There is a pair of segmental arteries at every intervertebral level (Plate 6).

They are as vital to the blood supply of the cord as the internal carotid and the vertebral arteries are to the brain.

In the thoracic and lumbar regions they are commonly known as the 'intercostal' and the 'lumbar' arteries; they arise from the posterior aspect of the aorta.

In the neck they arise from the branches of the subclavian artery, and are often duplicated on one or other side (Plate 7).

In the sacral zone, the lateral sacral arteries are their main source, with contributions from the middle sacral, ilio-lumbar and/or lowest lumbar arteries.

Their distribution is described below.

2: The distribution point of the segmental arteries is at the intervertebral foramen (Plate 8) (Dommisse, 1972a; 1974)

Segmental arteries are present at every level on both sides. They proceed directly to the intervertebral foramen appropriate to their level, where they divide into their terminal branches. The division takes place at the entrance to the foramen.

Minor branches supply nutrient vessels to the vertebral bodies and paravertebral muscles en route (Plate 9).

The major branches are for the supply of intra- and extra-spinal structures.

The intra-spinal structures include the spinal medulla, the membranes of the cord, the intraspinal sections of the segmental nerve roots, and the vertebral bodies. The extraspinal structures include the nerve roots, the autonomic nerve trunks and ganglia, the paravertebral

muscles and the posterior body wall. The latter, in the
thorax and abdomen, is supplied by the terminal
branches of the segmental vessels, respectively the
intercostal and lumbar arteries. The medullary feeder
arteries, which are of principal interest, arise at variable
levels (Figs. 3.1–3.16). Because of this variability, every
intervertebral foramen is a potential site of origin of an
anterior and/or a posterior feeder vessel. Accordingly,
the intervertebral foramen is a *vulnerable point* in the
system of arterial supply of the cord and should be
treated with caution during the course of surgical
procedures. It is also a point of maximal concentration
of blood vessels and one at which bleeding is likely to be
brisk from arteries and veins. Rough handling, heavy
retraction, plugging in the event of haemorrhage, and
the application of cautery at this level are threats and
should be avoided. Ischaemia with neurological deficits
could be precipitated in the event of involvement of a
major medullary feeder. Structures other than the spinal
medulla, in particular the segmental nerve roots and the
paravertebral muscles, could be involved in the same
manner. It follows that in anterior surgical approaches
to the spine, ligation of segmental vertebral arteries
should be carried out as close to the source of origin of
these vessels as possible. In the case of thoracic and
abdominal exposures, ligation should take place close
to the middle line. The collateral vessels, referred to
below under *The arterial circles of the spine,* will then
ensure the continued integrity of spinal cord circulation.

3: The cord is totally dependant upon three longitudinal arterial trunks

The anterior medial longitudinal arterial trunk of the
cord is continuous, from the level of the olivary nuclei
of the medulla oblongata, to the tip of the conus
medullaris. It occupies a position over the anterior
median sulcus, and deep to it is the anterior median
longitudinal venous trunk of the cord.

The postero-lateral longitudinal arterial trunks are
the counterparts of the former but are paired vessels
which are continuous over the same distance. They are
smaller vessels, they ramify frequently between the
posterior nerve rootlets and they can be seen in their
whole length only when the latter are divided and
retracted. They communicate across the middle line,

most abundantly at the level of the cervical and lumbar enlargements.

Communications between the anterior and the posterolateral longitudinal arterial trunks are scanty, and by means of small arteries and arterioles. The exception is at conus medullaris, where there is a constant cruciate anastomosis (Plate 10).

The anterior longitudinal truncal vessel is consistently of larger calibre in the cervical and the lower thoracic regions, at the levels of the two major ganglionic enlargements (see below under *Functional zones*). In the thoracic region, in that portion of the spinal cord which extends from about the third thoracic to the eight thoracic vertebrae, it is of smaller calibre than in any other section and in the adult has a diameter of approximately 350 μmm. The length of the cord over the same region is approximately 20 cm (8 in), and this long segment derives its entire supply for the ventral component (see below), from a vessel no greater than one third to one half millimeter in diameter. Clearly, interference with blood supply at this level is likely to prove critical (see also below under *Feeder vessels*).

The thoracic cord, at between T3/4 and T8/9 vertebral levels is thus seen to be a **vulnerable zone** in spinal cord circulation.

4: The circulation of the spinal medulla comprises a ventral and a dorsal component (Adamkiewicz, 1881, 1882; Kadyi, 1889; Bolton, 1939; Woollam and Miller, 1958; Turnbull, 1971)

The ventral component includes the anterior median longitudinal arterial trunk, the anterior medullary feeders, the anterior perforating vessels of the median sulcus and the perforating pial vessels of the cord (Figs. 3.1–3.12; Plates 1, 2, 13, 14, 15).

The dorsal component includes the paired postero-lateral longitudinal arterial trunks, the posterior medullary feeders and the perforating pial vessels (Figs. 3.13–3.14; Plates 3, 4).

The anterior arterial system supplies approximately the anterior two thirds and the posterior system supplies the posterior one third of the cord (Suh and Alexander, 1939). Communications between the anterior and posterior arterial components of cord supply are scanty, except only at the distal extremity where arterial circles cross the lateral surface of the conus medullaris (Plate 10). Arteriolar and capillary communications form only tenuous surface links between the three longitudinal trunks in the cervical and the thoracic regions (Plate 4). The absence of capillary anastomoses within the substance of the spinal medulla has been consistently recorded.

5: The longitudinal arterial trunks are supplied by feeder vessels at proximal, collateral and distal levels
The main supply of the longitudinal arterial trunks of the cord is from the collateral medullary feeder arteries. Their frequency and variable levels of incidence are indicated in Figures 3.1–3.16.

They represent the persistent few of those vessels which, during the growth and development of the neural tube, occur at every segmental level (Woollam and Millen, 1958), and they are concentrated at the zones of ganglionic enlargement.

Proximally, the longitudinal trunks receive consistent support from the anterior and posterior spinal arteries (Plates 1, 2, 3).

Distally, the support which the longitudinal trunks receive from various possible sources is of a more equivocal nature. A substantial medullary feeder arising in the lumbar or sacral region, distal to the conus medullaris, is of frequent occurence. It may be for the reinforcement of either the anterior or the postero-lateral trunk. In addition, the main trunks may derive support one from the other, through the medium of transverse communications between the anterior and the posterior trunks on the one hand (Plate 10), and between the postero-lateral trunks on the other (Plate 4). The matter is more fully discussed below under *The direction of flow in the blood vessels.*

A further interesting facet is the support which the thoracic cord receives from the longitudinal arterial trunk in the cervical and lumbar regions. The arteries are smaller and the medullary feeders are less numerous in the thoracic region which is, with justification, referred to as 'an arterial watershed' (Suh and Alexander, 1939) (Plate 12).

An overall predominance of anterior medullary feeders on the left side is recorded in this series, and a curious right-sided predominance in the cervical zone only.

An overall predominance of posterior medullary feeders on the right side is noted. These are facts which are presented without comment. (See below under the regional zones.)

6: The arterial supply of the grey matter is greater than the white matter

Woollam and Millen (1958), declared 'The poorest grey matter is indeed supplied with half as much again as the richest white matter'. The reason 'is a matter for speculation. Vascular density . . . has been correlated . . . (with a number of) factors indicating that the more metabolically active the area the better is its blood supply'. (Figs. 13, 17a, b).

The features of the longitudinal arterial trunks bear witness to this principle, for they are greatest in the cervical and lumbar zones of ganglionic enlargement (Figs. 4.1a, b, 6.1a, b) and least in the thoracic cord where the white matter of the longitudinal tracts predominates (Fig. 5.1a, b). By the same token, the central perforators of the anterior median sulcus are larger (up to 200 μmm), and most numerous (up to 10 per cm of cord length), in the cervical and lumbar zones. (Figs. 4.1a, b, 6.1a, b). Microangiographic studies (Figs. 5.1a, b, 6.1a, b) serve to illustrate the comparative vascularity.

The comparative diameters of the longitudinal vessels at different levels are indicated in the diagrams (Figs. 3.1–3.14).

7: There are three main functional zones of the spinal cord

1. The cervical cord which includes the cervical enlargements. The latter extends from C3 to T1 segmental level (Fig. 4.1a, b).
2. The thoracic cord which extends from T2 to T12 segmental levels (Fig. 5.1a, b).
3. The lumbar cord which includes the lumbar enlargement and the sacral ganglia. It extends from L1 to S5 segmental levels, and it occupies the spinal canal from T9 to L2 vertebral levels (Fig. 6.1a, b).

Recognition of the three zones is important because of the interposition of the relatively poorly vascularised thoracic zone between the cervical and lumbar enlargements, and because of the threat it imposes to the central connections of the lumbar enlargement. Wolman (1965) in a series of 95 autopsies in spine-injured, plegic deaths demonstrated the presence of ischaemic lesions, which were associated with central necrosis of the cord.

8: The medullary feeder arteries of the cord display patterns of extreme variability

An average number of eight anterior feeders has been observed in this and in other series (Kadyi, 1889; Suh and Alexander, 1939; Woollam and Millen, 1958), and a range of from 2–17 which was reported by Woollam and Millen (1958), has been corroborated in the present study.

The posterior medullary feeders are smaller and more numerous, with an average of 12, and a range of from 6–25. Six cadavers in the present series have been examined for both anterior and posterior medullary feeders, and in them no formula has been determined by which the anterior pattern may be calculated on the basis of a known posterior pattern, or *vice versa*.

Again, a single feeder in the cervical area may enjoy the support of only one feeder elsewhere, or of many. In cadaver 3247 (Fig. 3.1) there were two anterior feeders only, located at T2 level on left and at T8 level on the right side. When these factors are considered, then there are three deductions:

1. There can be no 'safe area' in spinal cord circulation. It follows that when surgical procedures are planned, an approach to the spine which circumvents the site of origin of the medullary feeders at the intervertebral foramen (Plate 8), is mandatory.
2. That at the thoracic cord (which extends from T2/3 to T8/9 vertebrae), the medullary feeders are less numerous and more widely spaced than elsewhere, and that in this zone the cord is most vulnerable to noxious stimuli.
3. That in view of the total dependance of the cord on the longitudinal arterial trunks, surgical planning must be directed towards their preservation. It is significant that in the thoracic region the anterior longitudinal trunk is consistently narrower than in the cervical and lumbar areas. It seldom exceeds a diameter of 250 μmm in neonates and 500 μmm in adults (Figs. 3.1–3.12, 3.15), (pp. 23–34, p. 37).

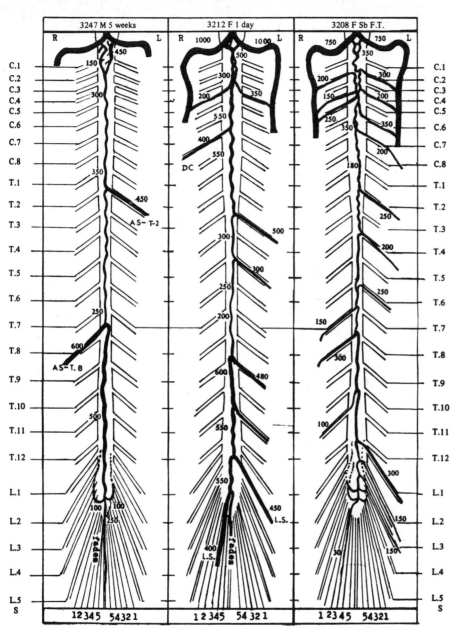

V.A. Vertebral artery. D.C. Deep cervical artery. S.I. Superior Intercostal artery. L.S. Lateral sacral artery.
Where not specially indicated, the source of supply is from the aortic segmental artery at the appropriate
level. Sb. denotes stillborn. F.T. denotes full-term.
Unit of length: micrometers.

Fig. 3.1   The anterior median longitudinal arterial trunk of the spinal cord in three neonatal cadavers.

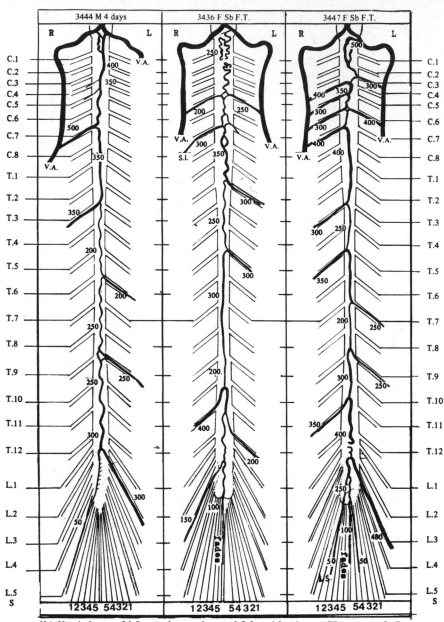

V.A. Vertebral artery. S.I. Superior Intercostal artery. L.S. Lateral Sacral artery. Where not specifically indicated, the source of supply is from the aortic segmental artery of the appropriate level.
Sb. denotes stillborn. F.T. denotes full-term.
Unit of length: micrometers.

Fig. 3.2   The anterior median longitudinal arterial trunk of the spinal cord in three neonatal cadavers.

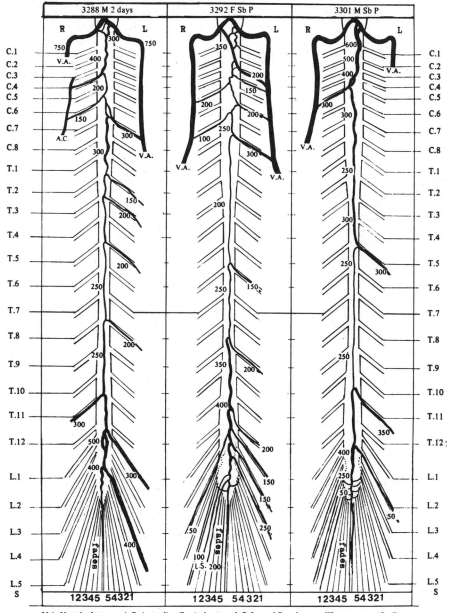

V.A. Vertebral artery. A.C. Ascending Cervical artery. L.S. Lateral Sacral artery. Where not specifically in-
dicated, the source of supply is from the aortic segmental artery of the appropriate level.
Sb. denotes stillborn. P. denotes prematurity. F.T. denotes full-term.
Unit of length: micrometers.

Fig. 3.3 The anterior median longitudinal arterial trunk of the spinal cord in three neonatal cadavers

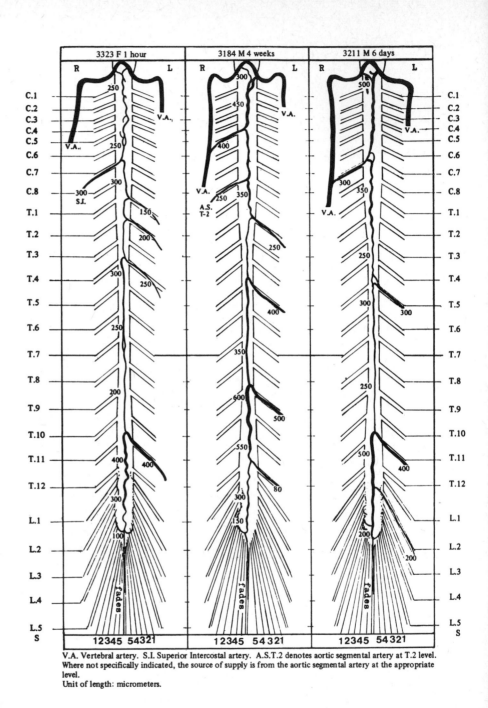

V.A. Vertebral artery. S.I. Superior Intercostal artery. A.S.T.2 denotes aortic segmental artery at T.2 level.
Where not specifically indicated, the source of supply is from the aortic segmental artery at the appropriate level.
Unit of length: micrometers.

Fig. 3.4 The anterior median longitudinal arterial trunk of the spinal cord in three neonatal cadavers

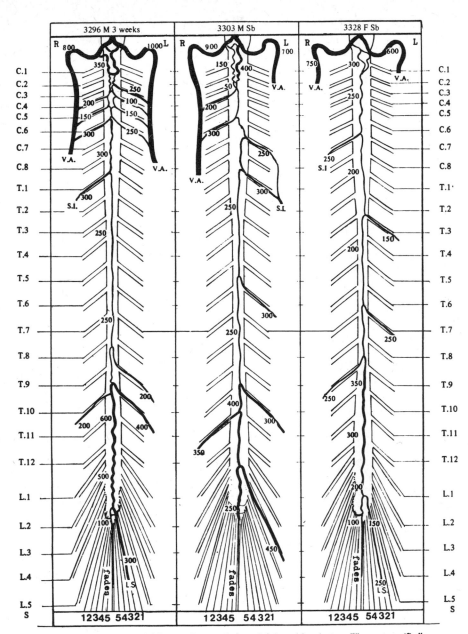

V.A. Vertebral artery. S.I. Superior Intercostal artery. L.S. Lateral Sacral artery. Where not specifically indicated, the source of supply is from the aortic segmental artery of the appropriate level.
Sb. denotes stillborn.
Unit of length: micrometers.

Fig. 3.5 The anterior median longitudinal arterial trunk of the spinal cord in three neonatal cadavers

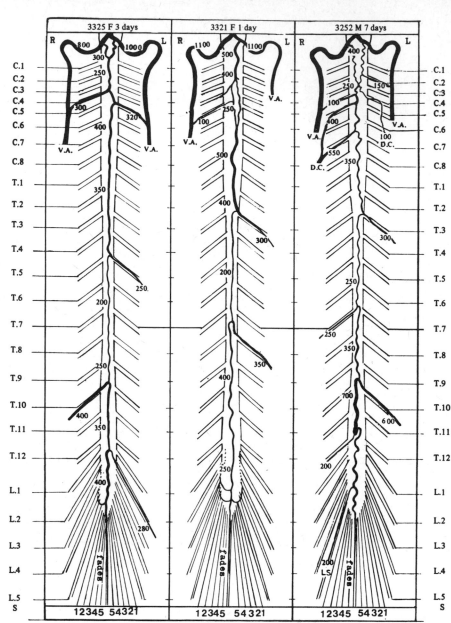

V.A. Vertebral artery. D.C. Deep Cervical artery. L.S. Lateral Sacral artery. Where not specifically indicated, the source of supply is from the aortic segmental artery of the appropriate level.
Unit of length: micrometers.

Fig. 3.6   The anterior median longitudinal arterial trunk of the spinal cord in three neonatal cadavers

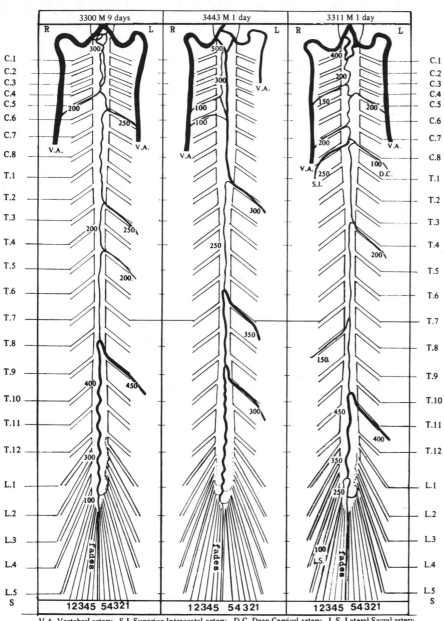

V.A. Vertebral artery. S.I. Superior Intercostal artery. D.C. Deep Cervical artery. L.S. Lateral Sacral artery
Where not specifically indicated, the source of supply is from the aortic segmental artery of the appropriate level.
P. denotes prematurity.
Unit of length: micrometers.

Fig. 3.7 The anterior median longitudinal arterial trunk of the spinal cord in three neonatal cadavers

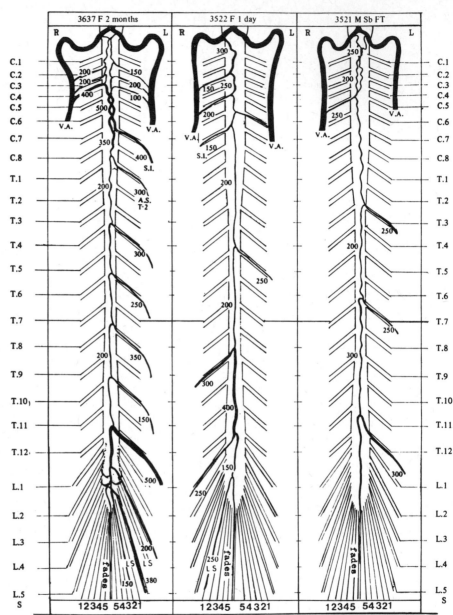

V.A. Vertebral artery. S.I. Superior Intercostal artery. A.S.T. 2 denotes the aortic segmental artery at T.2
level. Where not specifically indicated, the source of supply is from the aortic segmental artery of the
appropriate level.
Sb. denotes stillborn. F.T. denotes full-term.
Unit of length: micrometers

Fig. 3.8   The anterior median longitudinal arterial trunk of the spinal cord in three neonatal cadavers.

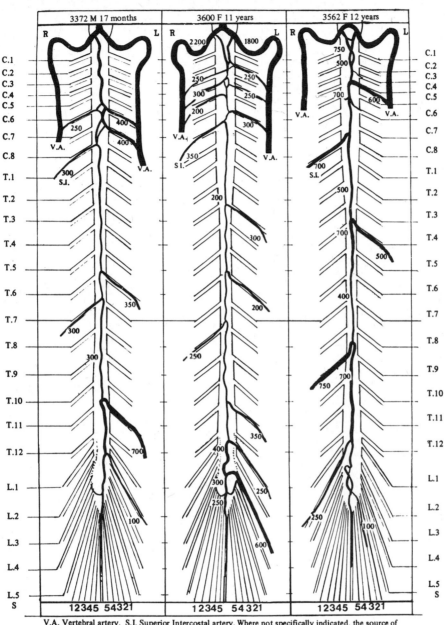

V.A. Vertebral artery. S.I. Superior Intercostal artery. Where not specifically indicated, the source of
supply is from the aortic segmental artery of the appropriate level.
Unit of length: micrometers.

Fig. 3.9   The anterior median longitudinal arterial trunk of the spinal cord in one infantile and two
early adolescent cadavers.

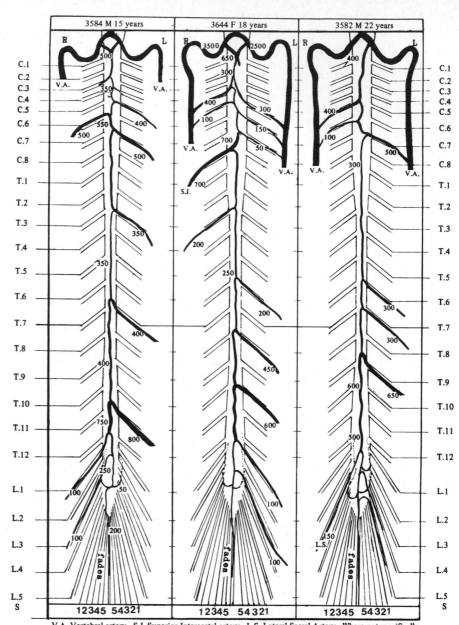

V.A. Vertebral artery. S.I. Superior Intercostal artery. L.S. Lateral Sacral Artery. Where not specifically indicated, the source of supply is from the aortic segmental artery of the appropriate level.
(Note: In specimen 3584 above, the source of the medullary feeders was not identified).
Unit of length: micrometers.

Fig. 3.10   The anterior median longitudinal arterial trunk of the spinal cord in two adolescent and one adult cadavers.

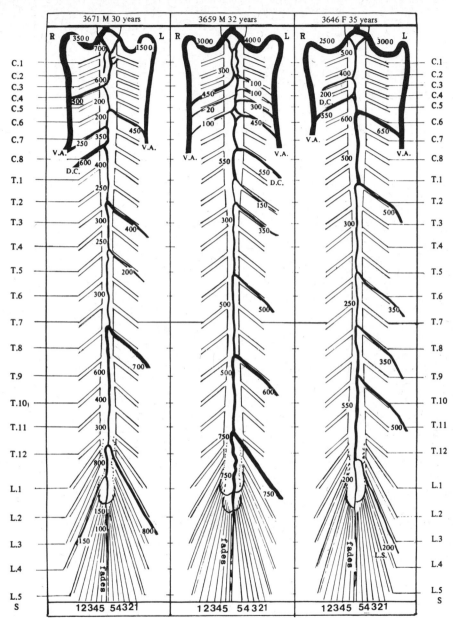

V.A. Vertebral artery. D.C. Deep Cervical artery. L.S. Lateral Sacral artery. Where not specifically indicated, the source of supply is from the aortic segmental artery of the appropriate level.
Unit of length: micrometers.

Fig. 3.11 The anterior median longitudinal arterial trunk of the spinal cord in three adult cadavers.

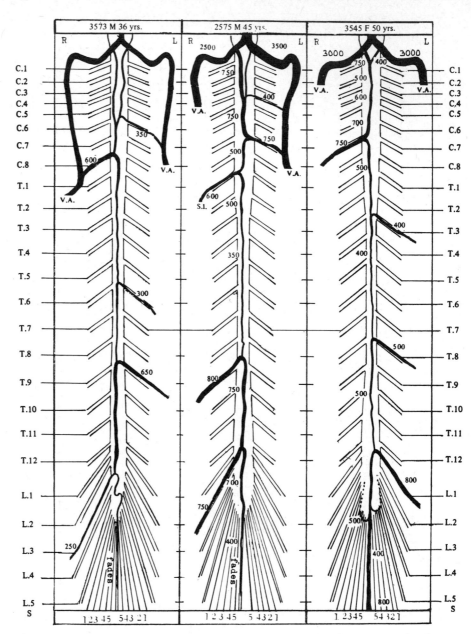

V.A. Vertebral artery. S.I. Superior Intercostal artery. Where not specifically indicated, the source of supply is from the aortic segmental artery of the appropriate level.
Note: In specimen 3545 above, the source of the medullary feeders was not identified.
Unit of length: micrometers.

Fig. 3.12   The anterior median longitudinal arterial trunk of the spinal cord in three adult cadavers.

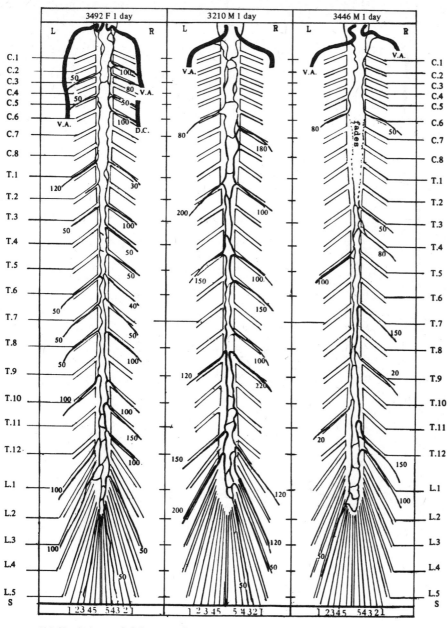

V.A. Vertebral artery. D.C. Deep cervical artery.
Unit of length: micrometers.

Fig. 3.13 The postero-lateral longitudinal arterial trunks of the spinal cord in three neonatal cadavers.

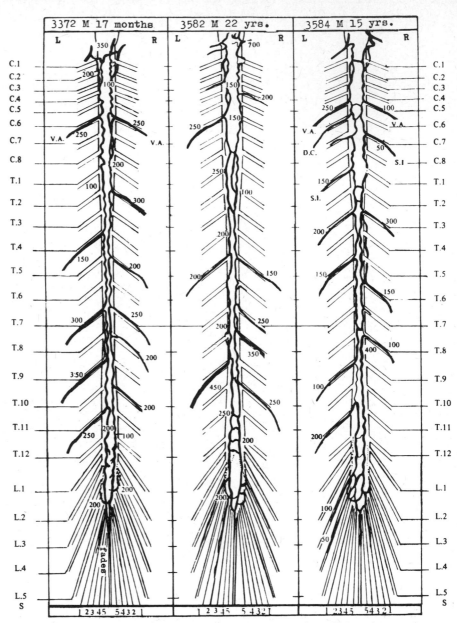

V.A. Vertebral artery. D.C. Deep cervical artery. S.I. Superior intercostal artery. The posterior communicating vessels are well illustrated at the conus.
The approximate size of the vessels is indicated in micrometers.

Fig. 3.14 The postero-lateral longitudinal arterial trunks of the spinal cord in one infantile, one **adolescent** and one adult cadaver.

THE ANTERIOR MEDULLARY FEEDERS OF THE SPINAL CORD
Their frequency at each level in 36 human cadavers at from neonatal to adult stages.

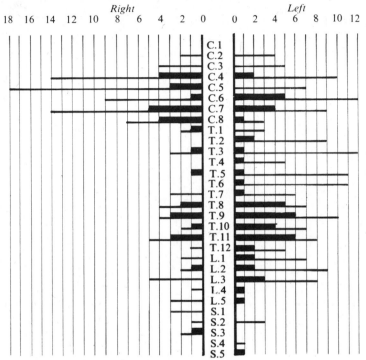

Large medullary feeders are indicated by a thick line.
A large feeder in the neonate is one with a diameter not less than 350 micrometers, and in the older age groups, not less than 450 micrometres.
The artery of Adamkiewicz is included in the above group.

Fig. 3.15 **The anterior medullary feeder arteries of the spinal cord. Their frequency and levels of incidence in 36 cadavers.**

THE POSTERIOR MEDULLARY FEEDERS OF THE SPINAL CORD
Their frequency at each level in 12 cadavers.

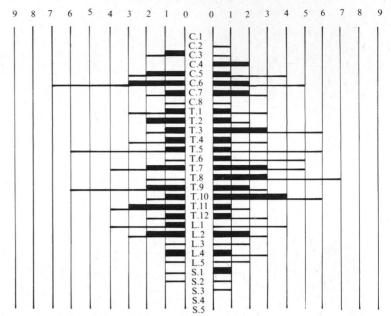

Vessels with a diameter of 200 micrometres or greater are indicated by a thick line.

Fig. 3.16 The posterior medullary feeders of the spinal cord. Their frequency in 12 cadavers.

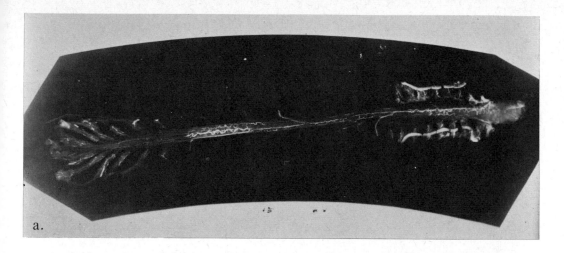

a.

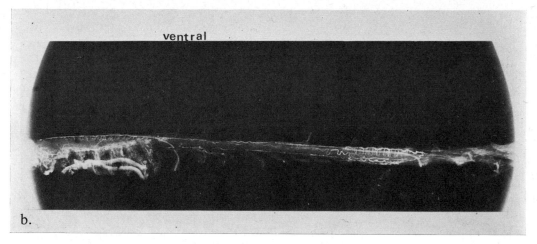

ventral

b.

Fig. 3.17 Microangiogram of a spinal cord excised from a neonatal cadaver. a. Antero-posterior view, showing also the medulla oblongata and the vertebral arteries. b. Lateral view.

9: The direction of blood flow in the longitudinal arterial trunks

The direction of flow is controversial, and deductions arising from the injection of contrast medium are unreliable. Woollam and Millen (1958) comment: '(it is) tempting although quite unjustified . . . to speculate as to the direction of flow in the arterial system on the results of the injection of cadavers'.

The conformation and the angle of entry of tributaries of the longitudinal trunks provide more reliable information.

Proximally, the anterior and the posterior spinal

arteries arise from the vertebral arteries (or their branches), and become continuous with the longitudinal trunks into which, presumably, they direct their contents (Plates 1, 3).

Collaterally, the medullary feeders form T, Y or inverted U junctions beyond which the flow of blood may take place in a proximal or a distal direction, or in both directions simultaneously (Plate 2).

Distally, at conus medullaris level, the medullary feeders join the longitudinal trunk by means of inverted U junctions; favouring a caudally directed flow but permitting also the opposite, for the benefit of the thoracic cord (Plate 2).

At the lumbar level, the picture is complicated by the communicating vessels on one or both sides of the conus medullaris, which form a link between the anterior and posterior arterial systems (Plate 10). In them, the direction of flow is equivocal and, while generally believed to be in an antero-posterior direction, may be postero-anterior. Romanes (1965) presents the case for the latter postulate and declares: 'In the coccygeal part of the spinal cord there is a large communication between the anterior and posterior spinal arteries, and at this level the anterior spinal artery is suddenly reduced to a small vessel on the conus and filum terminale. The above communications, which are usually symmetrical but which may be present on one side only form the largest communication between the three longitudinal arteries at any level of the spinal cord. Between the entry of the great spinal artery (the artery of Adamkiewicz), and the origin of these communicating branches, the anterior spinal artery remains of uniform calibre despite the number of branches arising from it, and this suggests the possibility that the communicating branches transmit blood to the anterior from the posterior spinal arteries, a possibility supported by the fact that large feeding vessels on the dorsal roots in the lumbar region send their major branches caudally'.

Fried *et al.* (1970) conducted *in vivo* studies on experimental animals and observed the direction of the flow of a blue dye in the blood stream, under certain stringent conditions. The concept of a constant direction under all circumstances would however seem sterile for just as in the circle of Willis at the base of the brain, so also in the vessels of the cord, the direction of flow is reversible and the arterial circles of the cord provide those 'substitution pathways', which were described by Lazorthes *et al.* (1971).

The arterial inflow is thus seen to consist of the medullary feeders which are supported by a series of arterial circles. In the author's view already expressed elsewhere (Dommisse, 1972a, 1974a), the three longitudinal trunks may 'be regarded as the innermost portion of a complicated 'arterial circle' which although more extensive and more complicated than the circle of Willis at the base of the brain, functions in terms of identical principles and permits of a reversibility of flow and of alterations in the volume of flow, in response to . . . metabolic demands. . . .'

On the other hand, the arterial outflow from the feeder system of vessels is through the central, sulcal and the pial perforating vessels of the cord. They are numerous and are described by Woollam and Millen (1958) as follows: 'There are about 200 central (sulcal perforating) branches in all, that is, one to every 2 mm of spinal cord. In the human there are about eighty in the thoracic region, forty-five in the cervical region, thirty-five in the lumbar region and twenty-five in the sacral region. Their density is, however, at its lowest in the thoracic region and at its greatest in the cervical and lumbar enlargements of the cord' (Plates 13, 14, 15).

In order to maintain a constant flow at the perforating 'outlet points', a constant and adequate hydrostatic pressure is necessary within the system. The longitudinal arterial trunks are seen in this study to constitute just such 'hydrostatic chambers', in which the pressure and the in- and out-flow are the vital factors. The direction of the in-flowing circulation is a variable factor which is so adjusted as to ensure the filling of the whole length of the longitudinal channels at all times and under all circumstances. In this manner, the neuronal tissue of the cord is ensured against ischaemia, and an instant collateral circulation is called into action when the definitive vessels are threatened. The cord is able to withstand anoxia for no longer than two or three minutes. An instant collateral system of supply is essential for survival.

9: The arterial circles of the cord (Plates 16–19)
(Dommisse, 1972a)
The arterial circles which serve the cord and which offer

'substitution pathways' (Lazorthes *et al.*, 1971) for the filling of the medullary feeders are extensive and abundant throughout the length of the vertebral column, from basi-occiput to coccyx. They extend also laterally to involve the various branches of the subclavian artery and the external carotid artery in the neck, and the aortic segmental arteries in the thoracic and lumbar regions (see below).

The innermost arterial circles are placed in direct contact with the spinal medulla and consist of a series of arterio-arterial anastomoses (arterial circles or loops or arcades), which form links between various trunks and their branches and serve as alternative pathways for the maintenance of spinal cord circulation. Anterior medullary feeders from the left and right vertebral arteries are linked by the anterior median longitudinal trunk (Plate 16).

The postero-lateral longitudinal trunks display arterial circles at all levels, in the form of transverse communications (Plate 4). They are richest where the need is greatest, at the cervical and lumbar enlargements. The vessels on the one side lend support to those of the other.

The second set of arterial circles of the spinal cord is within the extra-dural space of the spinal canal, encircling the dural sac with arteries of varying size. In the cervical region, a fairly constant set of transverse arterial links traverses the extra-dural space, anterior to the dural sac at each vertebral level. In the neck they are of small calibre and are demonstrated only when filling of the vessels has been adequate. In the thoracic region they are vessels of substantial size (Fig. 3.18), and in the middle line they offer numerous nutrient arteries which gain the substance of the vertebral bodies by passing through the posterior longitudinal ligament and entering the nutrient foramina. There are transverse and longitudinal arterial circles, some of them offering alternative pathways to the segmental arteries from which the medullary feeder arteries take origin, including the artery of Adamkiewicz (Plate 17).

A third set of arterial circles occurs in the extra-vertebral tissue planes, at many levels. They link the segmental arteries of the two sides by means of loops which pass from one side to the other, and deep or superficial to the anterior longitudinal ligament of the spine (Plates 18, 19).

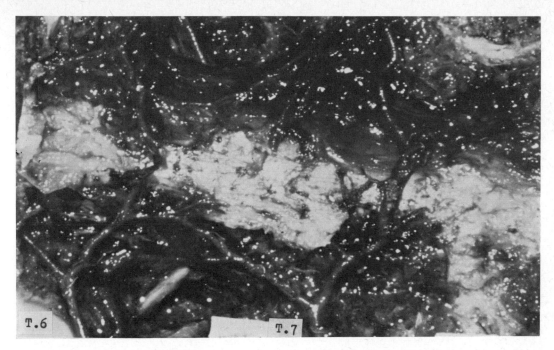

Fig. 3.18 Microdissection in mid-thoracic region, showing an arterial circle crossing transversely in the extradural space and linking the two segmental arteries.

They occur more laterally also, and in the neck they sometimes (60 per cent of cadavers) form links between the branches of the subclavian and the external carotid arteries. In them, branches of the ascending pharyngeal artery communicate freely and form arterial circles with branches of the vertebral and of the ascending cervical artery (Fig. 3.19).

In the thoracic and the lumbar region, the circles are completed at variable levels by branches of the segmental arteries which arise at the inter-vertebral foramina and which proceed proximally, distally and transversely (Fig. 1.1).

In order that a larger field and one in depth might be visualised, the technique of examination was supplemented by angiographic studies. The arterial circles at the conus medullaris were well displayed (Plate 10), and the radiographic picture of the postero-anterior communications at the conus medullaris served to complement the microphotograph of the dissected vessels in the same region (Fig. 6.1a, b).

Arising from these findings, it is postulated that the arterial circles of the spinal cord serve the same purpose for the medulla as the circle of Willis serves for the brain. It provides an effective safeguard against ischaemia and necrotic myelitis.

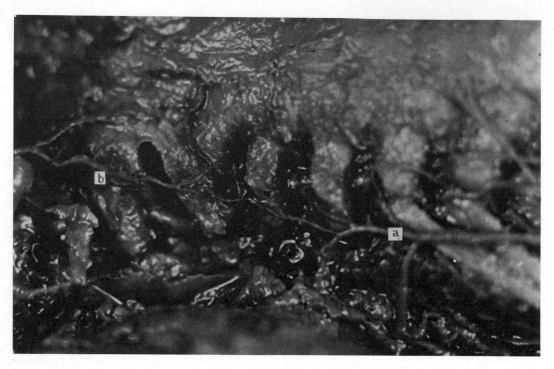

Fig. 3.19   The neck extra-vertebral arterial circles connecting branches of the ascending cervical arteries (a) and the ascending pharyngeal arteries (b).

4. The Cervical Zone of the Spinal Cord

In this report, the term 'cervical cord' refers to the cervical neural segments together with the first thoracic segment, and it includes the ganglionic enlargement of the brachial plexus. It extends to the level of the first thoracic vertebra and in the adult it is about 10 cm long. It makes up about 22 per cent of the length of the entire spinal medulla.

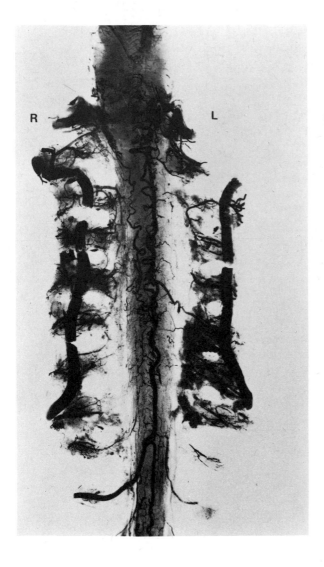

Fig. 4.1 Microangiogram of cervical cord vessels in a neonatal cadaver (enlarged)
a. antero-posterior view

The cervical cord enjoys a rich circulation, in conformity with the principle which governs the arterial supply of grey and of white matter (Fig. 4.1a, b principle 6, p. 21).

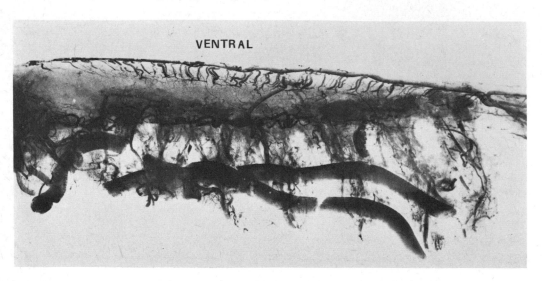

VENTRAL

Fig. 4.1　Microangiogram of cervical cord vessels in a neonatal cadaver (enlarged). b. lateral view.

The anterior median longitudinal arterial trunk of the cord is frequently duplicated from its proximal portion, distally for a variable number of segments, as far as C6 but seldom further (Plate 1). This feature is a persistence of the embryonic vessels which on both sides are the longitudinal links between the segmental arteries of the developing neural tube (Streeter, 1918; Woollam and Millen, 1958; Patten, 1968).

The anterior spinal arteries, the collateral cervical medullary feeders, and the more distal part of the longitudinal trunk itself, each contribute in greater or lesser measure to the continued filling of the cervical portion of the longitudinal channel. This was demonstrated in cadaver 3436 (Figs. 2.1, 4.2), in which, although the truncal vessel was discontinued at C2/3 level (Fig. 4.2), circulation was maintained from proximal and distal sources and the cord presented a normal, healthy appearance. This specimen focusses attention on direction of flow in the longitudinal arterial trunks of the cord. Clearly, in this instance blood flowed distally in the proximal segment of the vessel and proximally in the distal segment. Equally

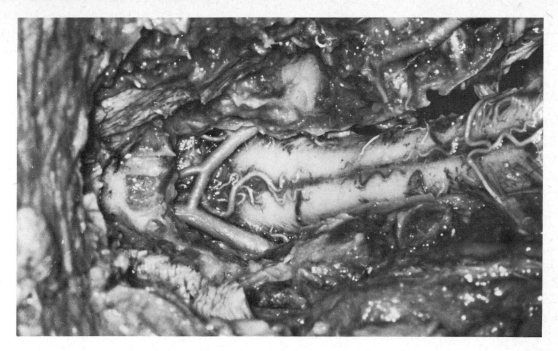

Fig. 4.2 The anterior median longitudinal arterial trunk is discontinuous at about C2/3 level. An unusual variant.

clearly, the flow of blood was directed at maintaining
cord circulation at all levels, through the medium of the
'outlet points' (Principle 9, p. 39), which are the
anterior perforators of the median sulcus.

The anterior medullary feeder arteries have been
dissected in detail, with the aid of the binocular surgical
microscope, in every instance in thirty-six human
cadavers. The findings have been recorded in respect of
the number, size, levels of incidence and source of origin
(Tables 4.1, 4.2).

The posterior feeders in eighteen human cadavers have
been studied and recorded in the same manner as above
(Tables 4.4, 4.5).

A summary of the tabulated findings in the series is as
follows:

TABLE 4.1

THE ANTERIOR MEDULLARY FEEDER ARTERIES OF THE CERVICAL CORD THEIR SIZE AND LEVELS OF INCIDENCE IN 36 HUMAN CADAVERS

SPECIMEN	AGE	SEX		SEGMENTAL LEVEL (RIGHT)								SEGMENTAL LEVEL (LEFT)								Total per case
		M	F	C2	C3	C4	C5	C6	C7	C8	T1	C2	C3	C4	C5	C6	C7	C8	T1	
3447	Sb FT		F			400	300	300	400				300			400				6
3444	4 days	M							500											1
3436	Sb FT		F		200		200		300						250					3
3637	2 mos		F	150		400							200	100	250	250	400		300	8
3521	Sb FT	M		200	150															1
3522	1 day		F				200	100	150							250				4
3443	1 day P	M				100	100													2
3300	9 days	M					200							100		250				2
3311	1 day	M				150			200			150				250				5
3252	7 days	M				150	400		550	250								100		5
3321	1 day		F			100	100													1
3325	3 days		F			300									320					2
3328	Sb		F			300			250										300	1
3303	Sb	M				200	150	300			300		250	100	150		250			4
3296	3 wks	M				200		300	400					350		250				8
3212	1 day P		F			200			300											3
3211	6 days	M																		1
3247	5 wks	M																		0
3208	Sb FT		F	200		150	250		300	250		300		200		350	200			7
3184	4 wks	M					400		300	250										2
3323	1 hr		F																	2
3301	Sb P	M					300												150	1
3292	Sb P		F				200		100				200	150		200	300	300		6
3288	2 days	M				300		150	100		300									3
3584	15 yrs	M						500	750						400	500	500			3
3545	50 yrs		F				550								300					1
3646	35 yrs		F		200	450	20	100								550		550		3
3659	32 yrs	M				450		100					100	100		450				8
2576	48 yrs	M						250		300	600			400			750			3
3372	17 mos	M				600	400			700						400	400			4
3562	12 yrs		F											600						2
3582	22 yrs	M						100								400	500			3
3573	36 yrs	M							350	600						350				2
3600	11 yrs		F	250	250	300	200							250		300	50			7
3644	18 yrs		F			400	100			700					300	150				6
3671	30 yrs	M				500			250	600						450				4
TOTAL 36		20	16	2	4	14	18	9	14	7	2	4	5	10	7	13	9	3	3	124

The approximate size of each feeder artery is indicated in terms of micrometres.
Sb denotes stillborn.   FT denotes full-term.   P denotes prematurity.

TABLE 4.2

THE ANTERIOR MEDULLARY FEEDER ARTERIES OF THE CERVICAL CORD
THEIR DERIVATION AND LEVELS OF INCIDENCE IN 34 HUMAN CADAVERS

SPECIMEN	AGE	SEX M	SEX F	R C2	R C3	R C4	R C5	R C6	R C7	R C8	R T1	L C2	L C3	L C4	L C5	L C6	L C7	L C8	L T1	Total per case
3447	Sb FT		F			VA		VA	VA				VA			VA				6
3444	4 days	M							VA											1
3436	Sb FT		F	VA			VA		SI											3
3637	2 mos		F		VA	VA							VA		VA		SI		T2	8
3521	Sb FT	M			VA	VA														1
3522	1 day		F		VA	VA	VA		SI							VA				4
3443	1 day P	M					VA	VA												2
3300	9 days	M				VA	VA							VA		VA				2
3311	1 day	M				VA			VA	SI				DC	VA			DC		5
3252	7 days	M					DC		VA			VA								5
3321	1 day		F				VA													1
3325	3 days		F			VA			SI						VA					2
3328	Sb FT		F						SI											1
3303	Sb FT	M				VA	VA	VA	DC				VA	VA	VA	VA				4
3296	3 wks	M				VA		VA	VA				VA	VA		VA				8
3212	1 day		F																	3
3211	6 days	M												VA		VA				1
3247	5 wks	M																		0
3208	Sb FT		F	VA		VA	VA	VA	SI	T2		VA		VA		VA	SI			7
3184	4 wks	M							SI		SI									2
3323	1 hour		F				VA	VA												2
3301	Sb P	M							VA											1
3292	Sb P		F				VA		VA	DC		VA	VA	VA		VA	VA	VA		6
3288	2 days	M				AC		AC					VA				VA	VA	SI	3

SPECIMEN	AGE	SEX M	SEX F	R C2	R C3	R C4	R C5	R C6	R C7	R C8	R T1	L C2	L C3	L C4	L C5	L C6	L C7	L C8	L T1	Total per case
3646	35 yrs	M			DC	VA	VA	VA					VA	VA	VA	VA	VA		DC		3
3659	32 yrs	M				VA	VA	VA			SI			VA		VA	VA			8
2575	48 yrs	M						VA						VA	VA	VA	VA			3
3372	17 mos	M								SI	SI			VA		VA	VA			4
3562	12 yrs		F				VA	VA												2
3582	22 yrs	M				VA	VA			VA						VA	VA			3
3573	36 yrs	M			VA	VA	VA		SI			VA		VA		VA	VA			2
3600	11 yrs		F		VA	VA	VA		SI	SI						VA		DC		7
3644	18 yrs		F			VA	VA		VA	VA					VA	VA	VA	VA	SI	6
3671	30 yrs	M							VA	VA	DC					VA	VA	VA		4

SPECIMEN	AGE	SEX M	SEX F	R C2	R C3	R C4	R C5	R C6	R C7	R C8	R T1	L C2	L C3	L C4	L C5	L C6	L C7	L C8	L T1	Total
TOTAL 34		18	15	2	4	14	18	8	13	7	2	4	5	10	6	13	8	3	3	120

VA denotes vertebral artery.
AC denotes ascending cervical artery.
Sb denotes stillborn.

SI denotes superior intercostal artery.
T2 denotes Aortic segmental artery at T-2 level.
FT denotes full-term.

P denotes prematurity.
DC denotes deep cervical artery.

49

TABLE 4.3

**THE NUMBERS AND POSITIONS OF THE SIGNIFICANT MEDULLARY FEEDER
ARTERIES IN THE CERVICAL CORD AS NOTED BY DIFFERENT OBSERVERS**

	ANTERIOR RADICULAR ARTERIES	POSTERIOR RADICULAR ARTERIES
Adamkiewicz (1881)	Usually 3; at C4, C5 and C8	1 or 2; at C6 or C7
Kadyi (1889)	Usually 2; between C4 to C7; most commonly at C5 or C6	1 or 2; between C4 and C7
Suh and Alexander (1939)	1 or 2 in lower and 1 in upper cervical region, usually between C3 to C6	—
Bolton (1939)	—	A large one at C4
Zülch (1954)	1 or 2 usually at C6 or C7	—
Woollam and Millen (1958)	1 major at C6 or C7; 3 to 5 minor at segments above C6	1 at C2; 1 to 3 between C5 to C7
Gillilan (1958)	At least 2; larger one at C5 or C6, the next one at C3; almost never at C8	—
Perese and Fracasso (1959)	1 to 5 may occur at all levels; maximum between C3 to C7	—
Chakravorty, (1969)	2 or 3 may occur at any level, mostly between C4 to C6; very rarely at C8	1 or 2 may occur at any level between C2 to C6; usually one at C4

This table is reproduced with acknowledgement of B. G. Chakravorty (1969), Department of Surgery, University of Calcutta, and to the Editor, The Annals of the Royal College of Surgeons, England. *Ann. Roy. Col. Surg. Eng.,* **45**, 232–251. 1969.

THE ANTERIOR CERVICAL MEDULLARY FEEDERS

The number of feeder vessels varied from nil to eight in
this series and the average number was 3.4 per cadaver.
There was a right-sided preponderance of 4:3. The
breakdown in number per cadaver was:

Anterior cervical feeders	No. of cadavers
0	1
1	7
2	7
3	7
4	4
5	2
6	3
7	2
8	3
Total	36

The above figures should be compared with those of
Chakravorty (1969), who summarised the findings
gleaned from eight earlier reports, and added his own
which differed in some respects from each of the others
(Table 4.3).

The size of the anterior feeders in all age groups is
indicated in Table 4.1 on page 48, and with very few
exceptions, they were substantial vessels. The average
outside diameter was 245 and 380 μm in the neonates
and the older age groups respectively.

The levels of incidence (Tables 4.1, 4.2; Figs. 3.15–3.17)
conform to the principle that the richest blood supply
is at the region of ganglionic enlargement.

Vertebral level	No. of Anterior feeders
C2	6
C3	9
C4	24
C5	25
C6	22
C7	23
C8	10
T1	5

The source of origin of the anterior cervical medullary
feeders was traced in 34 cadavers, and the findings
proved of considerable interest. The vertebral arteries

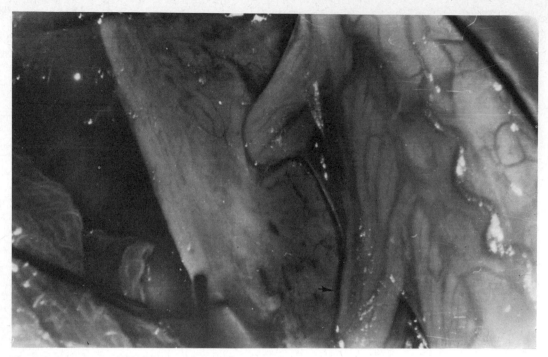

Fig. 4.3   Degenerative radiculopathy, as seen at operation.

were by far the most important source of supply and in fact, they dominated the picture. They supplied a total of 92 out of 120 anterior feeders, that is, 77 per cent in the series. The costo-cervical trunk, through its deep cervical and superior intercostal branches, supplied 24 feeders or 20 per cent, while the ascending cervical and the superior thoracic aortic segmental arteries supplied only two each (Table 4.2).

When attention was focussed on the thoracic inlet, then the position was reversed and the costo-cervical trunk was the most important supplier. It supplied no fewer than 21 out of a total of 36 anterior feeders at between C7 and T1 segmental levels. There were five from the deep cervical and sixteen from the superior intercostal artery. At these three levels, the vertebral artery contributed only thirteen (36 per cent), while the costo-cervical trunk contributed twenty one (58 per cent), and the superior thoracic aortic segmental artery only two (6 per cent).

It would appear that lesions at the thoracic inlet, with involvement of the costo-cervical arterial trunk,

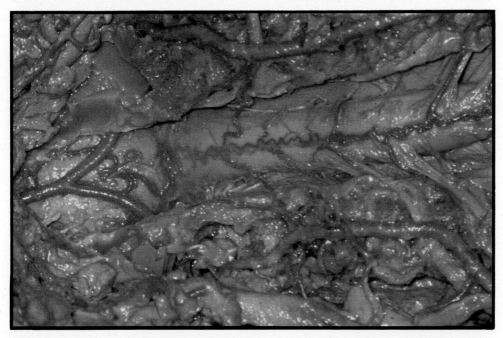

PLATE 1—The vertebral arteries, the anterior spinal arteries and the anterior median longitudinal arterial trunk of the spinal cord in the cervical zone.

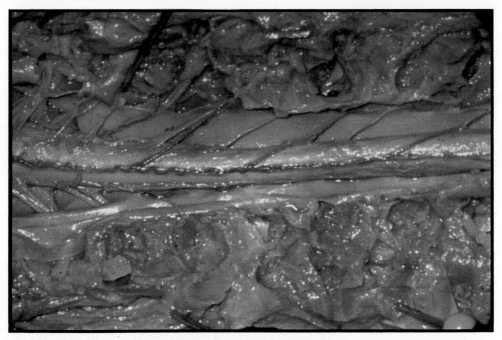

PLATE 2 (a) The anterior median longitudinal arterial trunk of the spinal cord. (In the thoracic zone. There are medullary feeder arteries at T2, T4 and T6 on left).

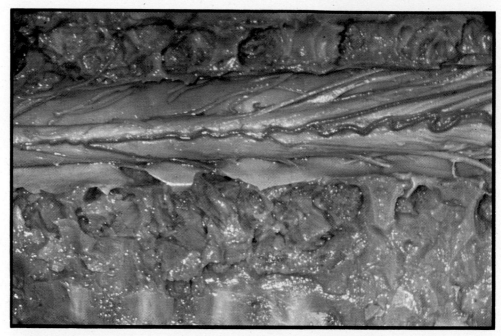

PLATE 2 (b) The anterior median longitudinal arterial trunk of the spinal cord. (In the lumbar zone. There are medullary feeder arteries at L1, L2, L3 on left and T11 on right, and the artery of Adamkiewicz is at L1 on the left side).

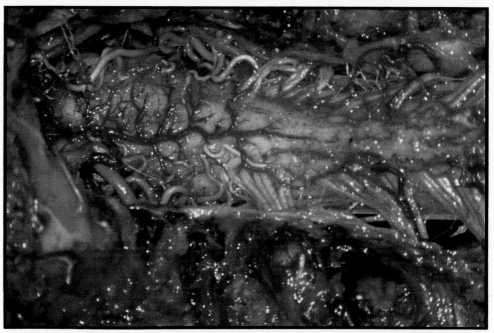

PLATE 3—The posterior aspect of the medulla oblongata and the upper cervical cord. The posterior spinal arteries are from the posterior inferior cerebellar arteries.

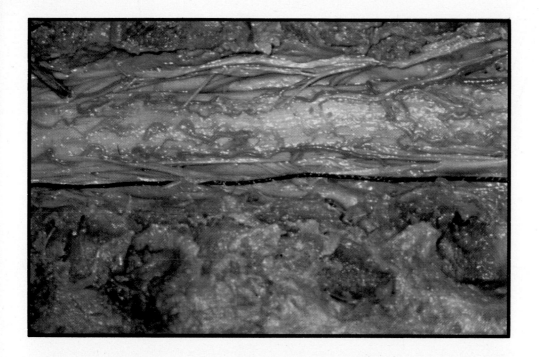

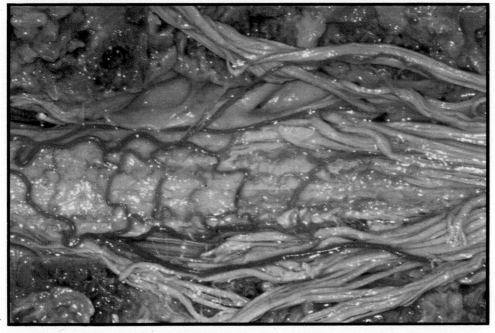

PLATE 4—The postero-lateral longitudinal arterial trunks of the spinal cord. (a) In the thoracic zone. (b) In the lumbar zone.

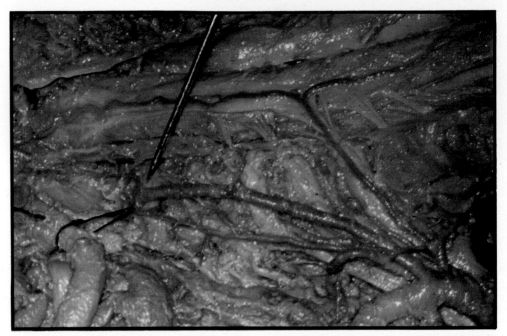

PLATE 5—A radicular artery and a medullary feeder artery, arising from the superior intercostal artery. They are separate entities.

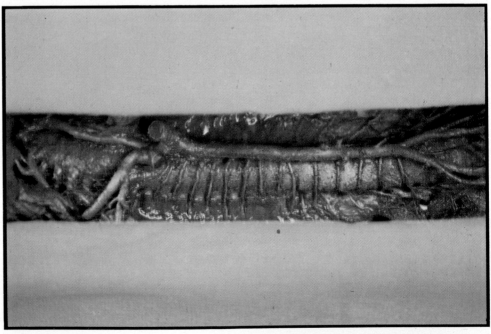

PLATE 6—The segmental vertebral arteries in the thoracic and lumbar regions arise from the aorta. In the neck they arise from branches of the subclavian artery.

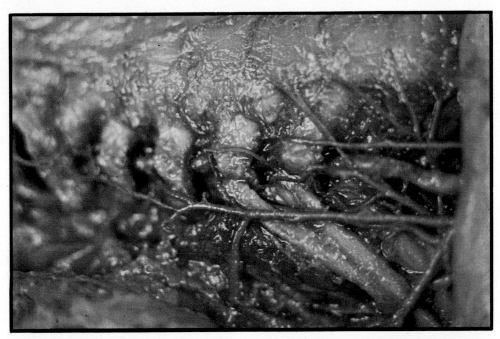

PLATE 7—The cervical segmental vertebral arteries arise from branches of the subclavian artery. There is an anastomotic link with branches of the external carotid artery in about sixty per cent of specimens.

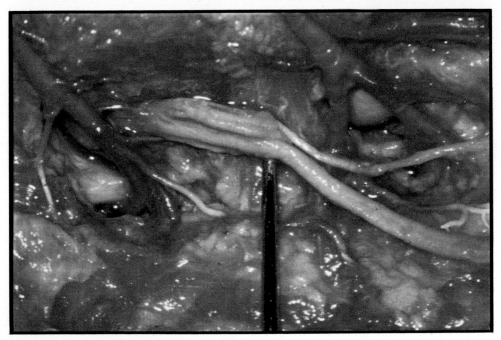

PLATE 8—The ARTERIAL DISTRIBUTION POINT of the segmental vertebral arteries, at the intervertebral foramen (L.1–L.2 levels show here).

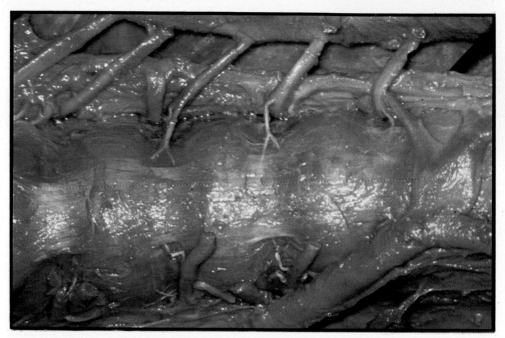

PLATE 9—Nutrient vertebral arteries arising from the aortic segmental arteries.

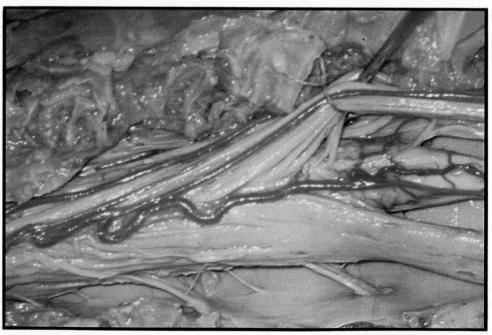

PLATE 10—The cruciate anastomosis at conus medullaris, between the anterior and posterior arterial vessels of the cord.

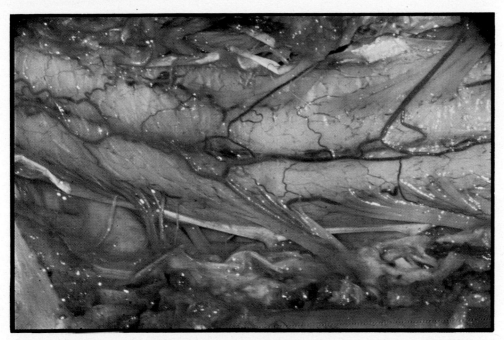

PLATE 11—Small anterior transverse, pial vessels in the cervical region, which anastomose with similar branches from the postero-lateral arterial trunks.

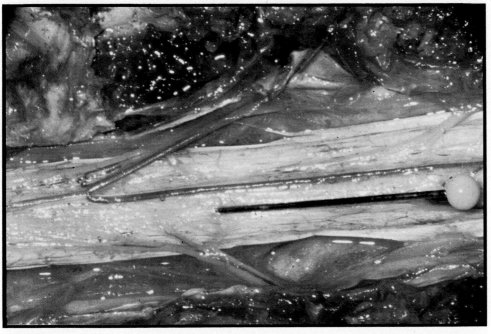

PLATE 12—The arterial 'watershed' of the anterior vessels of the cord, at mid-thoracic level, a critical vascular zone.

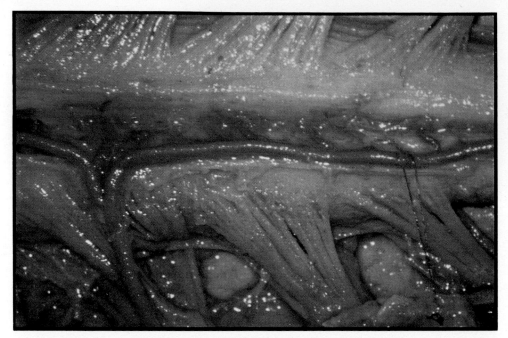

PLATE 13—The anterior sulcal perforating arteries of the spinal cord at cervical level.

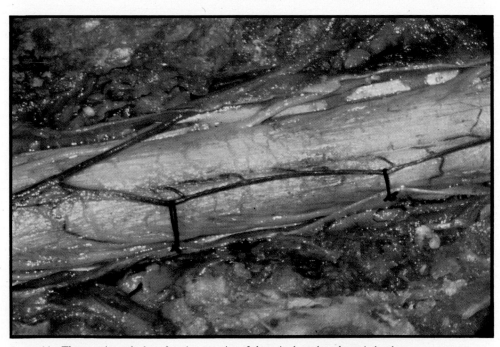

PLATE 14—The anterior sulcal perforating arteries of the spinal cord at thoracic level.

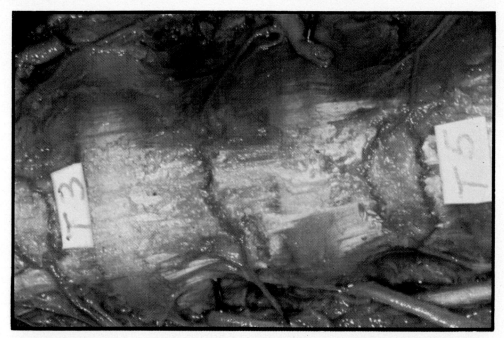

PLATE 19—Arterial circles in the extra vertebral tissue planes, linking the segmental arteries of opposite sides.

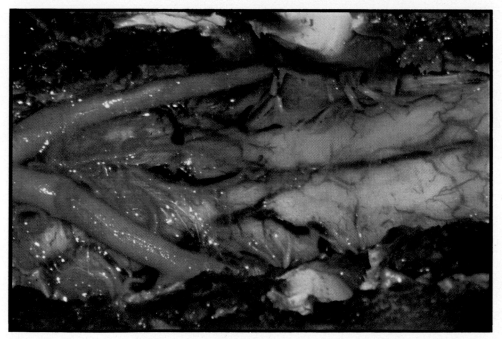

PLATE 20—The anterior longitudinal venous trunk of the spinal cord in the cervical region. It is deep to the artery.

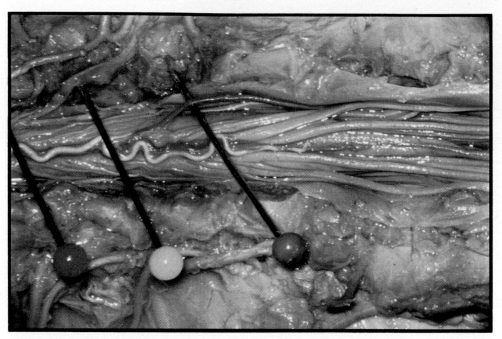

PLATE 21—The anterior longitudinal venous trunk of the spinal cord at the level of the conus medullaris.

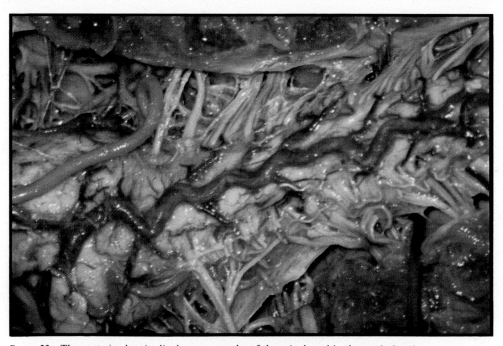

PLATE 22—The posterior longitudinal venous trunks of the spinal cord in the cervical region.

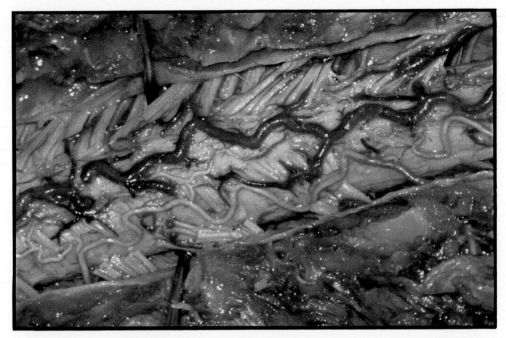

PLATE 23—The posterior longitudinal venous trunks of the spinal cord at the cervico-thoracic junction.

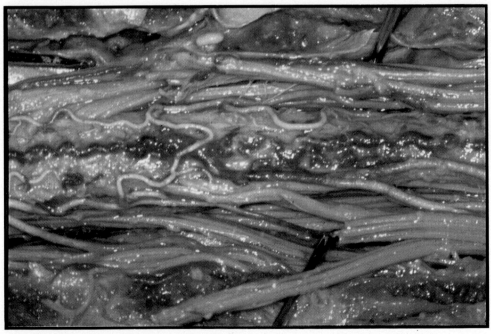

PLATE 24—The posterior longitudinal venous trunks of the spinal cord at the level of the conus medullaris.

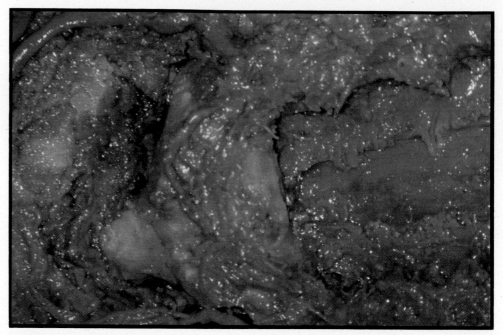

PLATE 25—The extradural component of Batson's venous plexus in the cervical region.

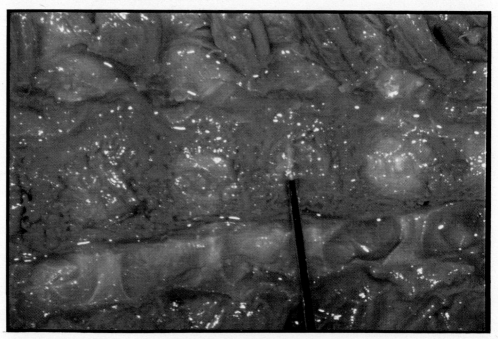

PLATE 26—The extradural component of Batson's venous plexus in the thoracic region.

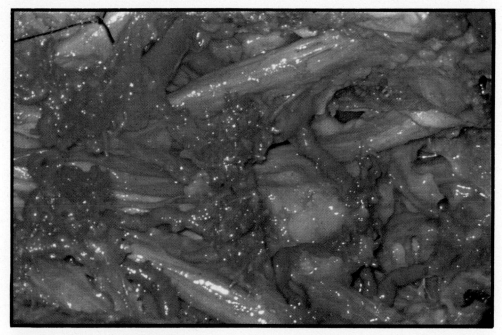

PLATE 27—The extradural component of Batson's plexus in the sacral region.

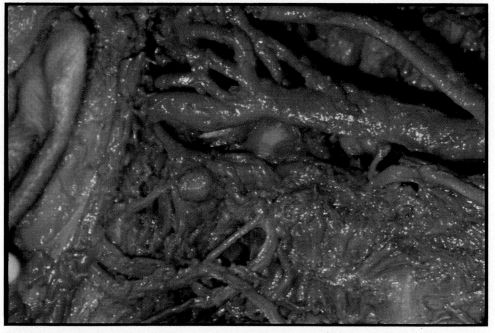

PLATE 28—Scalp veins and emissary veins of the skull, draining into the external jugular system and into the great confluence of venous sinuses at basi-occiput.

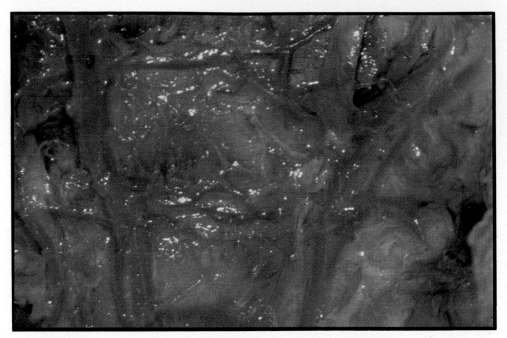

PLATE 29—The pre-sacral sympathetic trunks, with abundant nutrient vessels of supply.

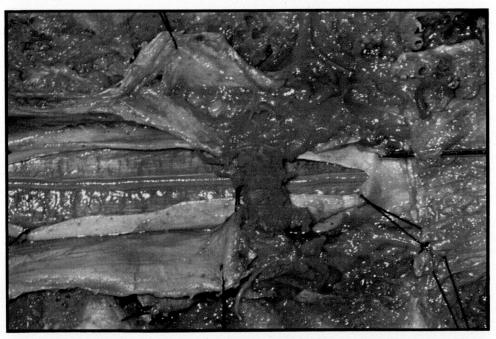

PLATE 30—The spinal cord at lumbar level. A thick, extradural membrane lines the inner surface of the spinal canal and contains portion of the extradural venous plexus within its layers.

could be associated with degenerative myelopathy due to relative or selective ischaemia of cord substance, and that neurological deficit of greater or lesser degree could result.

THE POSTERIOR CERVICAL MEDULLARY FEEDERS (Tables 4.4, 4.5)

The number of posterior feeders varied from nil to eight, and the average number was 2.9 per cadaver. They were equally distributed between left and right sides. The breakdown in number per cadaver was:

Posterior cervical feeders	No. of cadavers
0	1
1	2
2	7
3	3
4	2
5	1
6	1
7	0
8	1
Total	18

The size of the posterior feeders was generally little more than half of their anterior counterparts (Table 4.4), and the average outside diameter was 180 μm.

The levels of incidence of posterior cervical feeders were:

Vertebral level	No. of posterior feeders
C2	1
C3	3
C4	3
C5	9
C6	16
C7	8
C8	3
T1	9

The concentration of posterior vessels was at the region of the cervical ganglionic enlargement, and the principle governing the circulation in grey matter was upheld.

The source of origin of posterior cervical medullary feeders was traced in twelve cadavers, and the vertebral

TABLE 4.4

THE POSTERIOR MEDULLARY FEEDER ARTERIES OF THE CERVICAL SPINAL CORD
THEIR SIZE AND LEVELS OF INCIDENCE IN 18 HUMAN CADAVERS

SPECIMEN	AGE	SEX M	SEX F	SEGMENTAL LEVELS (LEFT) C2	C3	C4	C5	C6	C7	C8	T1	SEGMENTAL LEVELS (RIGHT) C2	C3	C4	C5	C6	C7	C8	T1	Total
3208	Sb FT		F						150	100								100	150	4
3323	1 hr		F							150	300									2
3292	Sb P		F					250								250				2
3443	1 dy P	M														100	250			2
3300	9 dys	M												100						1
3247	5 wks	M																		0
3296	3 wks	M							200		300						300			3
3637	2 mos		F					150								250			300	3
3492	1 day		F		80		50				120	100	80		50	100			30	8
3210	1 day	M						80								50				2
3446	1 day	M						80									180			2
3326	4 days	M					180		200							150				3
3457	Sb P		F												100					1
3254	1 day	M			200		250	250			300			200			300			6
3252	7 days	M					250	150			300				250					4
3372	17 mos	M						250								250				2
3584	15 yrs	M					250	150							100		250		300	5
3582	22 yrs	M						250						200						2
TOTAL 18		12	6	0	2	0	5	9	3	2	5	1	1	3	4	7	5	1	4	52

Sb denotes stillborn.　　FT denotes full-term.　　P denotes prematurity.
The approximate size of each feeder is indicated in terms of micrometres.

TABLE 4.5

THE POSTERIOR MEDULLARY FEEDER ARTERIES OF THE CERVICAL CORD
THEIR DERIVATION AND LEVELS OF INCIDENCE IN 12 HUMAN CADAVERS

SPECIMEN	AGE	SEX		SEGMENTAL LEVELS (LEFT)								SEGMENTAL LEVELS (RIGHT)								Total per case
		M	F	C2	C3	C4	C5	C6	C7	C8	T1	C2	C3	C4	C5	C6	C7	C8	T1	
3208	Sb FT		F						SI	AS T-2								SI	AS T-2	4
3323	1 hr		F							SI	AS T-2									2
3292	Sb P		F					VA								VA				2
3443	1 day P	M														VA	VA			2
3300	9 days	M												VA						1
3247	5 wks	M																		0
3296	3 wks	M					VA		VA		SI									3
3637	2 mos		F					SI									DC		AS T-2	3
3492	1 day		F		VA		VA				SI	VA	VA		DC	DC			SI	8
3372	17 mos	M						VA								VA				2
3584	15 yrs	M					VA	DC						VA	VA		SI			5
3582	22 yrs	M						VA			SI									2
TOTAL 12		7	5	0	1	0	3	5	2	2	4	1	1	2	2	4	3	1	3	34

VA denotes vertebral artery. SI denotes superior intercostal artery. DC denotes deep cervical artery. AS T-2 denotes aortic segmental artery at T-2 level.

Sb denotes stillborn. FT denotes full-term. P denotes prematurity.

artery supplied seventeen out of a total of thirty-four (50 per cent). The costo-cervical trunk, through its deep cervical and superior intercostal branches supplied thirteen feeders (38 per cent), and the superior thoracic aortic segmental artery supplied the remaining four (12 per cent). The deep cervical and the superior intercostal artery contributed four and nine posterior cervical feeders respectively.

At the thoracic inlet, which coincides approximately in level with the nerve roots of C7 to T1, the vertebral artery contributed two vessels only out of a total of fifteen, while the costo-cervical trunk together with the superior thoracic aortic segmental artery contributed thirteen (87 per cent). Once again, attention was focussed on possible lesions at the thoracic inlet which, if they involved the regional arteries could result in selective neurological deficit.

Radicular arteries for the supply of the nerve roots of the brachial plexus were large and numerous, and arose from two principal sources namely, the segmental cervical arteries peripherally (Plate 5), and the longitudinal arterial trunks of the spinal cord centrally (Plate 1).

Degenerative radiculitis (Fig. 4.3) as opposed to myelopathy was observed by Rossouw (1972) in the presence of thrombosis of a radicular artery.

5. The Thoracic Zone of the Spinal Cord

The thoracic cord includes the neural segments from the second to the twelfth thoracic levels and is devoid of ganglionic enlargement. It extends from the second to the ninth thoracic vertebrae and in the adult it is about 20 cm long, as compared with 45 cm for the entire medullary column. It makes up about 44 per cent of the length of the whole cord.

It receives a blood supply which is less abundant than the cervical and the lumbar regions, in conformity with the principle which governs the arterial supply of white matter (Fig. 5.1a, b; Principle 6, p. 21).

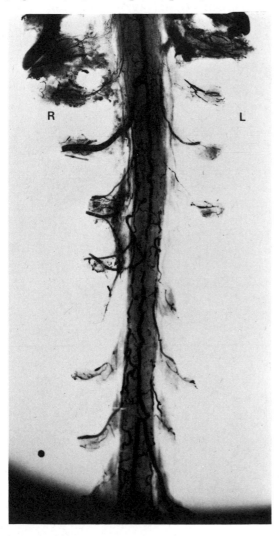

Fig. 5.1 Microangiogram of thoracic cord vessels in a neonatal cadaver (enlarged).
a. antero-posterior view.

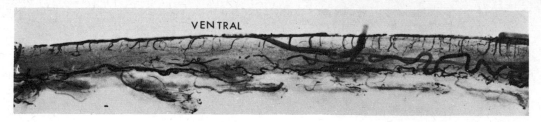

VENTRAL

b. lateral view—note small, infrequent anterior central perforating arteries.

The anterior median longitudinal arterial trunk of the cord is illustrated (Fig 3.1–3.12), each diagram being a reasonably accurate reproduction of the specimen represented. In the series of 36 cadavers, there was an almost uniform narrowing of the longitudinal vessel in that part of the cord which extends from the upper thoracic to just below mid-thoracic level. This was seen to be the critical vascular zone of the spinal cord, and it coincided with the zone of narrowing of the bony spinal canal (*see* Chapter 8).

In this region, the anterior sulcal perforating arteries (Plate 14) were of smaller calibre and lesser frequency than in the cervical and lumbar regions.

The anterior and posterior medullary feeder arteries have been dissected from origin to the point of distribution and have been found to arise from the aortic segmental arteries of the corresponding levels. It was noted however that the source of origin of the three most cephalad pairs of thoracic segmental arteries varied, and that the superior intercostal artery and the aortic thoracic segmental artery at T2 and T3 levels, were the main contributors. Individual patterns displayed wide variations.

The number, size and levels of incidence of the anterior and posterior thoracic feeders, and details of the three longitudinal arterial trunks are presented (Tables 5.1, 5.2; Figs 3.1–3.14).

THE ANTERIOR THORACIC MEDULLARY FEEDERS

The number of feeder vessels varied from one to five and the average number was 2.4 per cadaver. There was a left-sided preponderance of 4.7:1 in the series (Table 5.1).

The breakdown in numbers of feeders per cadaver was:

Anterior thoracic feeders	*No. of cadavers*
1	6
2	15
3	11
4	3
5	1
	Total 36

The size of the anterior thoracic feeders is indicated in Table 5.1. The overall average measurement of the outside diameter of these vessels was 282 and 400 μm in neonates and older age groups respectively, and corresponded closely with those of the cervical region.

When both size and number of the anterior feeders in the two zones were considered, then it was clear that circulatory volume was relatively and absolutely inferior in the thoracic cord, which in this series received only 86 as compared with 124 feeder vessels. The cervical cord is only half as long as the thoracic cord, yet it receives a number of anterior medullary feeders which is half as great again as that of the latter. Once again the principle of greater vascularity of grey matter is demonstrated.

The levels of incidence.

Vertebral level	*No. of feeders*
T2	9
T3	15
T4	5
T5	12
T6	11
T7	9
T8	11
T9	14
	Total 86

The anterior feeder vessels in the thoracic area are distributed more or less uniformly and there is no local concentration of vessels. Although fewer in number than elsewhere, they nevertheless fulfil the important role of reinforcing and maintaining the longitudinal arterial trunk.

The source of origin of the thoracic feeder vessels was traced in most specimens, and it proved to be the thoracic aortic segmental arteries of the corresponding levels, with the exception of the two or three most proximal segments, where the superior intercostal artery was dominant (see Chapter 4).

THE POSTERIOR THORACIC MEDULLARY FEEDERS (Table 5.2)

The number of feeder vessels in this part of the cord varied from three to ten, and the average number in a series of twelve cadavers was 5.3 per cadaver. There was a right sided preponderance of 3:2, as opposed to the anterior feeders where a left-sided preponderance of 4.7:1 was recorded. There was no apparent relationship between the number of anterior and the number of posterior feeders in the individual cadaver, and no formula by which the number, size or level of incidence of one set of feeders could be deduced from a knowledge of the other. The breakdown in posterior feeders in the series was:

Posterior thoracic feeders	*No. of cadavers*
3	3
4	1
5	3
6	3
7	0
8	1
9	0
10	1
	Total 12

The size of the posterior thoracic feeders was approximately a half of their anterior counterparts (Table 5.2). The average outside diameter of the vessels was 153 μm, as compared with 320 μm and there were 5.3 posterior as compared with 2.4 anterior medullary feeders per average cord in the series.

The levels of incidence (Table 5.2).

The posterior feeders, like the anterior group, were fairly evenly distributed.

Vertebral level	No. of feeders
T2	4
T3	8
T4	6
T5	12
T6	6
T7	9
T8	10
T9	9

The source of origin of the posterior feeders was from the thoracic aortic segmental arteries, at the corresponding levels. At the thoracic inlet, the superior intercostal artery was the principal contributor.

TABLE 5.1

THE ANTERIOR MEDULLARY FEEDERS OF THE THORACIC SPINAL CORD
THEIR LEVELS OF INCIDENCE AND APPROXIMATE SIZE IN 36 HUMAN CADAVERS

SPECIMEN	AGE	SEX	R T2	R T3	R T4	R T5	R T6	R T7	R T8	R T9	L T2	L T3	L T4	L T5	L T6	L T7	L T8	L T9	Total
3447	Sb FT	F		300		350										250		250	4
3444	4 days	M		350											200			250	3
3436	Sb F.T.	F									300			300					2
3637	2 mos	F										250			250	250			3
3521	Sb FT	M											300				350		2
3522	1 day	F								300	300								2
3443	1 day P	M										250		250		350			3
3300	9 days	M											200	200				450	3
3311	1 day	M										300							1
3252	7 days	F							150			300							2
3321	1 day	F						250											1
3325	3 days	F												250		250	350		3
3328	Sb	F								250					300				2
3303	Sb	M												300				200	2
3296	3 wks	M										500		300					2
3212	1 day P	F																480	1
3211	6 days	M							600		450		200						3
3247	5 wks	M							300		250								2
3208	Sb FT	F						150			250			400				500	4
3184	4 wks	M									200		250	300					3
3323	1 hr	F													150				1
3301	Sb P	M															200		1
3292	Sb P	M																	
3288	2 days	M									150	200		200				200	4
3584	15 yrs	M									500	350				400	500		4
3545	50 yrs	F									150	400			350		350		4
3646	35 yrs	F										350						600	3
3659	32 yrs	M													500				4
2575	48 yrs	M						300							350				1
3372	17 mos	M								800			500						2
3562	12 yrs	F								750					300	300		650	2
3582	22 yrs	M																650	3
3573	36 yrs	M							250			300		300					2
3600	11 yrs	F		200											200				3
3644	18 yrs	F										400		200	200		450		3
3671	30 yrs	M															700		3
TOTAL 36		M 20 / F 16	0	3	0	1	0	3	4	4	9	12	5	11	11	6	7	10	86

The approximate sizes of the medullary feeders is expressed in micrometres.
The artery of Adamkiewicz is indicated by a thick horizontal underline.
Thoracic feeders are from aortic segmental arteries at corresponding levels.

TABLE 5.2

THE POSTERIOR MEDULLARY FEEDERS OF THE THORACIC CORD
THEIR LEVELS OF INCIDENCE AND APPROXIMATE SIZES IN 12 CADAVERS

SPECIMEN	AGE	SEX M	SEX F	LEFT T2	T3	T4	T5	T6	T7	T8	T9	RIGHT T2	T3	T4	T5	T6	T7	T8	T9	Total
3247	5 wks	M		200		100						100				100				3
3492	1 day		F	200				50	50	50	120			50	50	40	50	100	220	10
3210	1 day	M			50		150						50	80	100	50				8
3446	1 day	M					100										150	100	120	5
3326	4 days	M					180				250		50					180		3
3457	Sb P		F				60			150					30			150		5
3254	1 day	M							250		150		200	200			200		250	6
3252	7 days	M				200			150		150		250			250				4
3208	Sb FT		F								150				50			200		3
3582	22 yrs	M					200				450	300	200		150	150	250	350		5
3584	15 yrs	M			200	150	150				100				200			100		6
3372	17 mos	M							300								250	200		6
TOTAL 12		9	3	2	2	3	6	1	4	2	6	2	6	3	6	5	5	8	3	64

Sb denotes stillborn. FT denotes full-term. P denotes prematurity.
The approximate size of each feeder is indicated in terms of micrometres.

6. The Lumbar and Sacral Zones of the Spinal Cord

The study was continued from the cervical and the thoracic zones, to the most caudal aspect of the spine and to the distal extremities of the fifth sacral nerve roots. The same group of cadavers was used for each zonal study. The details of the incidence, levels, and size of the vessels are indicated in Tables 6.1 and 6.2.

The lumbar and sacral zone of the cord extends from the junction of the ninth and tenth thoracic vertebrae, to the conus medullaris at the middle of the first lumbar vertebra. It is about 15 cm in length in the adult, and

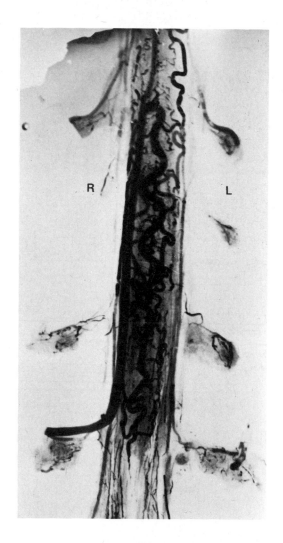

Fig. 6.1 Microangiogram of lumbar and sacral zones, with large and abundant vessels at anterior and posterior aspects (enlarged).
a. antero posterior view

makes up one third of the entire spinal medulla. In it
there are the lumbar and the sacral ganglionic
enlargements and accordingly, it enjoys a blood supply
which compares with that of the cervical enlargement
(Fig. 6.1a, b).

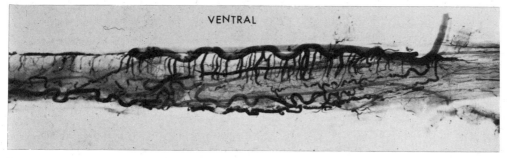

b. lateral view

The anterior median longitudinal arterial trunk of the
cord (Figs. 3.1–3.12) is largest in the lumbar and sacral
regions, and at the conus medullaris it communicates
with the posterior vessels via the cruciate anastomosis.

It is more tortuous in the neonate than in the adult
(*see* Chapter 7), and in the majority it tapers off and
ends on the filum terminale. Occasionally it is continuous
with a medullary feeder artery which joins it from a
distal (lumbar or sacral) level.

THE ANTERIOR LUMBAR AND SACRAL MEDULLARY FEEDERS

The number of feeders varied from nil to seven in the
series, and there was an average of 2.2 anterior feeders
per cadaver. There was a left-sided preponderance of
2:1. The breakdown was:

Anterior lumbar and sacral feeders	No. of cadavers
0	3
1	10
2	10
3	9
4	1
5	2
6	0
7	1
Total	36

The size of the anterior feeders is recorded (Table 6.1). The average outside diameter was 245 and 405 μm in neonates and the older age groups respectively.

Comparing the lumbar and sacral zones with the cervical, there was an advantage in favour of the cervical zone where the vessels were of closely comparable size, but were greater in number, in the proportion of approximately three to two.

The levels of incidence (Table 6.1):

Segment level	No. of feeders
T10	9
T11	13
T12	6
L1	9
L2	11
L3	13
L4	2
L5	4
S1–S3	9
S4–S5	2
Total	78

The source of origin was two-fold, namely the lumbar aortic segmental arteries at corresponding levels, and the lateral sacral arteries.

The latter are specifically indicated (LS), in Table 6.1 and it will be observed that a significant number of anterior feeders were from below the conus medullaris level and that they joined the anterior median longitudinal trunk from below, as compared with the thoracic and cervical feeders where they are from one or other side.

THE POSTERIOR MEDULLARY FEEDERS

The number of posterior feeders varied from 1–9 in the series and the average number was 4 per cadaver. There was a rightsided preponderance in the ratio of 7:5.

The breakdown in numbers per cadaver was:

TABLE 6.1

THE ANTERIOR MEDULLARY FEEDERS OF THE LUMBAR & SACRAL ENLARGEMENTS
THEIR LEVELS OF INCIDENCE, SOURCE AND APPROXIMATE SIZE IN 36 HUMAN CADAVERS

SPECIMEN	AGE	SEX		VERTEBRAL LEVELS (RIGHT)										VERTEBRAL LEVELS (LEFT)										Total
		M	F	T10	T11	T12	L1	L2	L3	L4	L5	S1-3	S4-5	T10	T11	T12	L1	L2	L3	L4	L5	S1-3	S4-5	
3447	Sb FT		F		350								50(LS)					300	480				250	4
3444	4 days	M									50													2
3436	Sb FT		F		400				150										200(LS)		380(LS)			3
3637	2 mos		F																		150(LS)			5
3521	Sb FT	M		150																				1
3522	1 day		F				250					250(LS)												2
3443	1 day P	M		300											400									1
3300	9 days	M																						0
3311	1 day	M				200						100(LS)		400										3
3252	7 days	M		600							200(LS)			600										0
3321	1 day		F	400																				1
3325	3 days		F															280				250(LS)		3
3328	Sb	M		300																				3
3303	Sb	M		300 / 400	350														450					3
3296	2 wks		F	200	250 / 400							400(LS)		250 / 400				450 / 150				300(LS)		2
3212	1 day P	M															750AS(L1)		200(LS)					0
3211	6 days	M																						5
3247	5 wks	M																						1
3208	Sb FT		F		100							80(LS)				80	300	150	150					1
3184	4 wks	M													400 / 350									2
3323	1 hr		F																					7
3301	Sb P	M															50	50						3
3292	Sb P		F						50		100(LS)	200(LS)				200	300	150	250					
3288	2 days	M			300										200					400				
3584	15 yrs	M					100							500	800		800					(LS)	500	3
3545	50 yrs		F					100																2
3646	35 yrs		F																					2
3659	32 yrs	M																						1
2575	48 yrs	M						750											200(LS)					1
3372	17 mos	M													700			100						2
3562	12 yrs		F				250		150(LS)						350		250							1
3582	22 yrs	M							250(LS)															1
3573	36 yrs	M															100							1
3600	11 yrs		F														250		600 / 100					3
3644	18 yrs		F											600			100	800						3
3671	30 yrs	M								150														2
TOTAL 36		20	16	2	5	1	2	2	5	1	3	6	0	7	8	5	7	9	8	1	1	3	2	78

LS Lateral Sacral Artery.

The letters in parenthesis which precede or follow a figure indicate the derivation. Where the derivation is not indicated, the medullary feeder arose from the lumbar aortic segmental artery. In a few instances, the source could not be identified because of incomplete filling with latex. The approximate size of the arterial feeders is indicated in micrometers.

Posterior lumbar and sacral feeders	No. of cadavers
1	2
2	3
3	1
4	2
5	0
6	1
7	2
8	0
9	1
Total	12

The size of the posterior feeders (Table 6.2).

The average overall size was 150 μm, and in the older age group, 225 μm.

Their source of origin was the same as the anterior medullary feeders. The cruciate anastomosis at the conus medullaris is between the anterior and the two postero-lateral longitudinal arterial trunks.

THE ARTERY OF ADAMKIEWICZ (Plate 17)

The 'arteria radicalis magna anterior' was described by Adamkiewicz (1881a, b) in the classic contribution. It is the largest anterior feeder 'in the upper lumbar portion of the cord', it occurs unilaterally and is usually on the left side.

In the computerised average version of the anterior medullary arteries presented by Suh and Alexander (1939), it is at T10 level on the left side.

In the present series, it occurred at from T7 to L4 levels, thus:

Vertebral level	No. of cadavers
T7	1
T8	2
T9	9
T10	5
T11	7
T12	2
L1	2
L2	2
L3	3
L4	1
Absent or indefinite	2
Total	36

TABLE 6.2

THE POSTERIOR MEDULLARY FEEDERS OF THE LUMBAR & SACRAL ENLARGEMENTS THEIR LEVELS OF INCIDENCE AND APPROXIMATE SIZES IN 12 CADAVERS

SPECIMEN	AGE	SEX M	SEX F	LEFT T10	T11	T12	L1	L2	L3	L4	L5	S1-3	S4-5	RIGHT T10	T11	T12	L1	L2	L3	L4	L5	S1-3	S4-5	Total
3247	5 wks	M		100				250						100										3
3492	1 day		F		100		100								150	100	150	200				50		7
3210	1 day	M				150		200									120		30	50		50		6
3446	1 day	M			200		180									150	100		120	50				4
3326	4 days	M										50								50				2
3457	Sb P		F	200			100					100		120		200	150				100			7
3254	1 day	M			150		300	150		300				200				250	120	200	50			9
3252	7 days	M									50											250		2
3208	Sb FT		F		200	200			150						200									4
3582	22 yrs	M												250										1
3584	15 yrs	M												250										1
3372	17 mos	M												200				80						2
TOTAL 12		9	3	2	4	2	4	3	1	1	1	2	0	6	2	3	4	3	2	3	2	3	0	48

Sb denotes stillborn. FT denotes full-term. P denotes prematurity.

The approximate size of each feeder is indicated in terms of micrometres.

It occurred on the left side in 28 cadavers (77 per cent) on the right side in 6 cadavers (17 per cent), and was absent or unidentified in 2 cadavers.

Kadyi (1889) reported the vessel at between T9 and L3 segment, and Suh and Alexander (1939) stated: '. . . it may be observed at any segment between T8 and L4'.

The positive identification of the vessel is not always possible and some of the difficulties are indicated in Tables 5.1 and 6.1, and also in Fig. 3.15, which reflects the incidence of large medullary feeders, comparable in size with the artery of Adamkiewicz.

The problems of identification included the following:

Cadaver 2575 (Fig. 3.12). There were two vessels of almost identical size, the first at T9 level on the right side (800 μm), and the second at L2 level on the right side (750 μm). Both qualify for the eponym.

Cadaver 3328 (Fig. 3.5). A vessel of 250 μm was present at T7 and S2 levels on left, and at T9 level on the right side. Each one of the three could qualify for the eponym.

Cadaver 3212 (Fig. 3.1). A vessel of 480 μm was present at T9 level on the left side, and one of 450 μm at L2 level on the left side. A third anterior vessel, 400 μm in diameter, was present at S3 level on the right side. Three great feeders serve the lumbar enlargement.

Romanes (1965) refers to the larger medullary feeders as 'great spinal arteries' and indicates their incidence in 22 human cadavers.

In the present series, 'a great spinal vessel' was regarded as one with a diameter of at least 350 μm in neonatal and at least 450 μm in the older age group. They are indicated in Fig. 9.6. There is a concentration of great vessels at the cervical and lumbar enlargements of the cord. The principle of a rich supply at the zones of ganglionic enlargement is constantly reaffirmed in this series.

In the thoracic region, great anterior vessels occur at all levels but in reduced numbers. In the lumbar zone there were 42 great anterior vessels in 36 cadavers, of which 34 were labelled as Adamkiewicz's artery. Those of slightly lesser dimensions resembled the former in all other respects and were presumably of equal significance.

In the cervical region, one or more anterior medullary feeders are usually found of a size comparable with the artery of Adamkiewicz.

In the course of surgical approaches to the spine, the relative significance of the artery of Adamkiewicz is a factor of prime importance. It may be present at any level from T7 to L4 on the left or the right side and it follows that care at each and every level is mandatory. When the level of the vessel has been identified pre-operatively, then care at that level and at every other level is still essential, for the preservation of the artery of Adamkiewicz at the expense of other anterior feeders cannot be regarded as a safeguard against ischaemia of the cord and neurological deficit.

7. A Comparative Study of the Blood Vessels of the Spinal Cord of Neonates and of Older Age Groups

Spinal cord circulation in neonates and in the older age groups is reported below. There were thirty neonatal cadavers, and twelve cadavers in age groups which varied from infantile to adult stages.

The similarities were more striking than the differences, and it was in the relative sizes of the blood vessels *vis-a-vis* the cord that the most important differences were detected. The patterns varied as widely in one series as in the other; the principles, on the other hand, were constant and identical.

The length of the cord *in situ* was measured from medulla to conus medullaris.

The weight and the volume of the cords of neonates and of older cadavers were recorded, after excision of cord with membrane. The results were as follows:

	Neonate	Older Group
Length of cord:	10–12.5 cm	40–50 cm
Weight of cord with membranes	7.0 g	91.0 g
Volume (displacement) with membranes	6.0 ml	79.2 ml

The average number and the range of variations of the medullary feeder arteries was determined:

	Neonate	Older Group
Average no. of anterior feeders	7.9	8.1
Range of anterior variations	2–17	4–16 (all age groups)
Average no. of posterior feeders	12.2	(all age groups)
Range of posterior variations	6–25	(all age groups)

The comparative numbers of anterior medullary feeders, and the average diameter of the anterior feeders were:

	Neonate	Older Group
1. Anterior cervical medullary feeders		
Average number	3.3	3.8
Average diameter	245 μm	380 μm

72

	Neonate	Older age group
2. Anterior thoracic medullary feeders		
Average number	2.3	2.5
Average diameter	282 μm	400 μm
3. Anterior lumbar medullary feeders		
Average number	2.3	1.8
Average diameter	245 μm	405 μm

The numbers, size, levels of incidence and source of origin of the anterior feeders in the various age groups are indicated in Tables 4.1, 4.2, 5.1, 6.1. The relative sizes of the anterior median longitudinal arterial trunk are indicated diagrammatically (Figs 3.1–3.12). The frequency of anterior feeders at each level in 24 neonatal and 12 older cadavers is indicated below.

THE ANTERIOR MEDULLARY FEEDERS OF THE SPINAL CORD
Their frequency at each level in 24 neonatal cadavers.

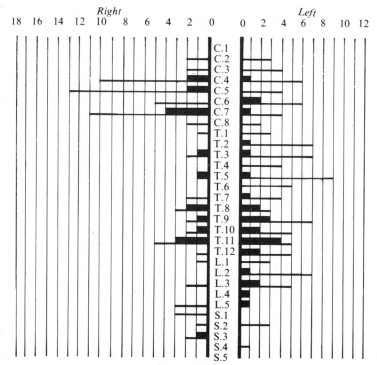

Large medullary feeders are indicated by a thick line.
A large feeder in the neonate is one with a diameter not less than 350 micrometers, and in the older age groups, not less than 450 micrometres.
The artery of Adamkiewicz is included in the above group.

THE ANTERIOR MEDULLARY FEEDERS OF THE SPINAL CORD
Their frequency at each level in 12 cadavers at ages from the infantile through the adolescent to the adult stages.

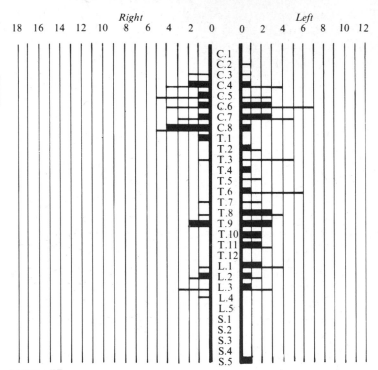

Large medullary feeders are indicated by a thick line.
A large feeder in the neonate is one with a diameter not less than 350 micrometers, and in the older age groups, not less than 450 micrometres.
The artery of Adamkiewicz is included in the above group.

The posterior medullary feeders were studied in a smaller series, of which only three were in the older age group. A comparison between the posterior feeders in the two age groups is offered in Tables 4.4, 4.5, 5.2, 6.2, and the conformation of the postero-lateral longitudinal arterial trunks is illustrated in Figures 3.13, 3.14.

The posterior medullary feeder arteries are smaller and more frequent than the anterior. The average diameters are approximately 150 and 325 μm respectively. Details of the actual sizes are reflected in Tables 4.4, 5.2, 6.2 for the posterior, and in Tables 4.1, 5.1, 6.1, for the anterior feeder arteries.

The average numbers of the posterior feeders *vis-a-vis* the anterior feeders in three zones of the cord were:

	Posterior feeders All age groups	Anterior feeders		
		All ages	Neonates	Older group
Cervical zone	2.9	3.4	3.3	3.8
Thoracic zone	5.3	2.4	2.3	2.5
Lumbar zone	4.0	2.2	2.3	1.8
Total	12.2	8.0	7.9	8.1

The diameter of the anterior median longitudinal arterial trunk in the different age groups is indicated in the diagrammatic representations of 36 spinal cords which are sub-divided into 12 groups (Figs 3.1–3.12).

Figures 3.1–3.8: Twenty-four neonatal cadavers.
Figure 3.9: One infantile and two early adolescent cadavers.
Figure 3.10: Two adolescent and one adult cadaver.
Figure 3.11: Three young adult cadavers.
Figure 3.12: Three adult cadavers at 36–50 years.

In every specimen, the anterior median longitudinal trunk is narrowest at about T6 segmental level, and in nearly every case, the narrowest section of the trunk extends over a total of four or five segments centred upon or close to T6 level.

Deviations from this rule (or principle), are rare and are accounted for by the presence of one or more large medullary feeders at or near T6 level (Cadaver 3562, Fig. 3.9).

In the cervical zone the anterior median longitudinal trunk is larger than in the thoracic zone, and sometimes it is duplicated. It is largest in the region of the lumbar enlargement and is generally about half as large again in the adult as in the neonate.

The anterior medullary feeders, too, are about half as large again in the adult with the exception of the lumbar zone where they are about twice as large (Table 6.1).

The postero-lateral longitudinal arterial trunks are illustrated (Figs. 3.13, 3.14), in three neonatal cadavers and in three cadavers of an older age group.

In each group, the general configuration of the postero-lateral longitudinal arterial trunks is the same, and each trunk is continuous from medulla oblongata to conus medullaris. They divide and deviate frequently and they communicate with each other at many levels.

They are covered in greater or lesser measure by the posterior nerve rootlets which must be divided and retracted for full exposure. It is presumed that reports of discontinuous postero-lateral longitudinal arterial trunks are due to this factor (Plate 4).

TORTUOSITY OF THE LONGITUDINAL ARTERIAL TRUNKS OF THE SPINAL CORD

In the neonate the longitudinal arterial trunks are tortuous (Plate 2). In the adult, they are less tortuous in some cadavers and straight in others (Plate 14).

The growth of the longitudinal channels from neonatal to adult stage is in length rather than in calibre, and in the adult they are four times as long as in the neonate, but only half as large again in respect of diameter. The perforating branches of the longitudinal trunks are concentrated into a relatively short area in the neonate, but are spread out over a wider area as the length of the cord increases and the tortuosity of the longitudinal arterial trunks diminishes. The metabolic demands of the neural tissue are greatest during growth, and are progressively reduced as growth slows down and the demands of function rather than growth are to be satisfied.

THE ARTERIAL CIRCLES OF THE SPINAL CORD

Arterio-arterial anastomoses or 'circles' were observed at all levels, in both the neonatal and the older age-group series.

They were undiminished in the adult, and the communications occurred across the middle line as well as between ipsi-lateral neighbours (Plates 18, 19). No significant differences in the age groups were detected.

8. The Width of the Spinal Canal

The spinal canal is of variable width and shape throughout its length. In the sacral region is is flattened from before backwards and there are wide tunnels for the passage of the roots of the cauda equina.

In the cervical region and also at the lumbar enlargement it is capacious, with a large lateral extension for each of the roots of the brachial and the lumbar plexuses.

In the thoracic region, the contrast is striking for it is here that the canal is narrowest and assumes the rounded or semi-elliptic shape of 'natural intention'. It is consistently narrowest in that part of the vertebral column which extends from T4 to T8/9 levels (Table 8.1), and occasionally to T10 or T11 level. The narrow zone of the spinal canal corresponds almost exactly with that part of the cord in which the blood supply is least profuse.

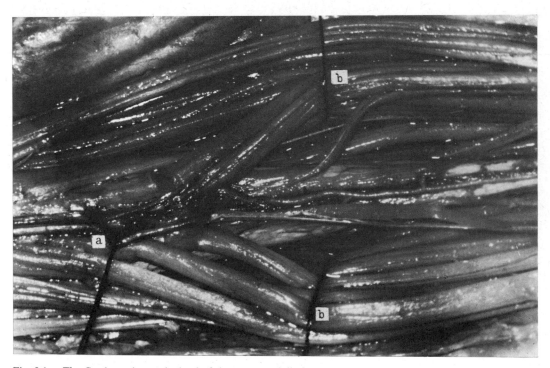

Fig. 8.1a   The Cauda equina at the level of the conus medullaris.

The examination of a series of six sets of macerated vertebral columns served to confirm the above radiological findings (Table 8.2).

Distal to the level of the conus medullaris, the lateral diameter of the spinal canal increases and the antero-posterior diameter decreases (Fig. 8.1a, b), as befits the cauda equina.

Vascular lesions of the roots of the cauda equina have hitherto not been described, but traction lesions resulting in peripheral nerve paralysis have recently been reported in pelvic fractures with subluxation of the sacro-iliac joint (Harris, 1973). The possibility of a vascular lesion of the nerve roots cannot be excluded. In these cases there has been good motor and poor sensory recovery of function.

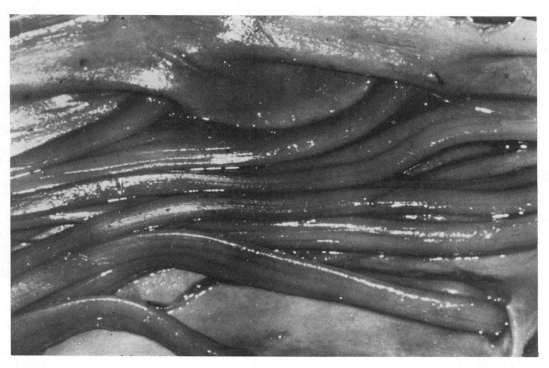

Fig. 8.1b   The Cauda equina distal to the conus. The spinal canal is wide in the lateral dimension, and flattened antero-posteriorly.

TABLE 8.1

THE CRITICAL NARROW ZONE

NAME	AGE	SEX	D1	D2	D3	D4	D5	D6	D7	D8	D9	D10	D11	D12	L1	L2	L3	L4	L5	SI
E.L.	4	M	21	19	17	16	15.5	15.5	16	16	16	17	17	17.5	20	20	20	22	24	
A.M.d.P.	14	F	23	20	18	17.5	17	16.5	16	16.5	17	18	20	Rotated			22	25	28	30
L.v.R.	15	F	23	22	20	18	18	19	19	19	19	20	23	Rotated			22	26	31	
M.G.	9	F	21	18	17	17	17	17	18	18.5	19	19	19	22	22	22.5	23	25	27	
J.L.	32	F	22	22	17	16	16	15	15	15.5	16	17	18	21.5	23	25	26	26	30	
B.A.L.	37	M	27	23	21	19	19	19	18	18.5	19	19	20	25	27	27	27.5	29	34	
J.G.	11	F	21	18	17	16.5	16.5	16	15.5	16.5	17	17	18	21	22	22	23	24		
M.R.B.	3	F	21	18	17	16	15.5	15.5	16	17	17.5	18	18	20	21	21	21	21	27	30
W.B.	18/12	M	18	18	15	14	15	15	15	15	15	15	16	18	19	19	19	21	25	
E.C.	35	F	23	21	20	19	19	18.5	18.5	19	20	21	22	25	26	26	26	26	32	
I.C.	42	M	?	22	21	21	21	21	22.5	23	24	25	28	32	32	30	31	33	34	
E.C.	11	F	23	20	19	18	17	17	17	18	18.5	19	21.5	25	25	25	26	26	?	
S.J.P.F.	11	M	24	20	19	17.5	17	16.5	16.5	16.5	16.5	16.5	17	19	21	22.5	24	25	27	
H.J.B.	27	M	?	?	20	19	19	19	18.5	19	20	20	21	26	26	26.5	27	27.5	30	
A.S.B.	68	M	23	22	21	20	18.5	19	19.5	19	19	19	20	23.5	25	25	28	31	?	
M.B.	68±	F			19.5	18.5	18	18	18.5	19	19.5	20	21.5	26	26.5	28	30	34	40	
G.M.	13	M	?	?	18	17.5	17	16.5	17	17.5	17.5	18.5	20	22.5	23.5	24	24	27	35	
A.C.	41	M	25	21.5	21.5	21	20	21.5	21	20	20	20	21	26	25	27	27	29		
D.F.C.	12	M	?	?	18.5	18	17.5	17.5	17.5	17.5	18.5	21	24	26	26.5	25	25	23.5		
V.A.C.	33	F	?	20	19	17.5	17	17	17.5	17.5	19	20	23	28	28	27	27	31	32	
K.L.	40	M	22	21	18	17	17	17	16	16	17	17	17	18	20	22	25	26	35	?
T.R.	35	F	23	20	18	17	16	16.5	16	16	16	17	18	21	21	22	23	25	30	?
J.C.F.	49	F	21	19	17	17	18	18	18	19	19	20			25					
L.H.F.	55	M	22	22	20	18	17	17	17	17.5	18	19	22	25	27	28	28			
W.D.	40	F	21	20	19	19	19	19	18	18	18	19	20	22	24	24	26			
J.D.	12	F	21	18	17	16	15	16	16	17	17.5	18	19	21	21	21	22			
T.J.D.	42	M	23	21	21	19	18	18.5	19	21	22	23	25	27	28		28			
A.D.	20	M	25	21	19	19	19	18	18.5	19	20	20	21	23	25	25	23			
C.D.	17	F	23	20	17	17	16	16.5	17	18.5	20	20	20.5	21.5	22.5	24	24			
M.D.	16	F	22.5	20	18	16.5	16.5	17	18	19	19	20	21	24	Rotated		24			
Y.J.	17	F	26	22	19	18	17	17	17	17	17.5	18.5	20	24	27	27	27			
R.H.	15	M	26	25	22	21.5	20	20	19	18.5	18	21	22	27	28	27	28			
M.N.	15	M	24	21	19.5	18.5	17.5	16.5	17	18	18.5	18.5	20.5	22.5	24	24	24.5			
R.S.	16	M	27	23	21	20	20	20	21	21	21.5	22	23	24	25	25	27			
F.W.L.B.	30±	M	32	26	23	22	20	20	20	19.5	20	22	22	24	28	28	29			
F.B.	63	M	26	22	19	18	17	17	16	17	16	17	18	22	23	26	26			
F.B.	2	M	16	15.5	15	15	14	15	16	16	16	17	19	19	19	20	20			
R.B.	15	M	23	20	17	16	16	16	15	16	17	17	18	20	21	21	22			
H.B.	16	F	22	19	17	16	15	15	15	16	17.5	19	21	21.5	22.5	26	27			
J.B.	5	F	21	19	17.5	16	15.5	16	16.5	17	17	18	20	22	22	22	22	24	27	
H.M.	4	M	21	18	17	16.5	16.5	16.5	16	16.5	16.5	17	19	21	23	22	23	24	25	?
A.M.V.	17	F	22	19	18	15	16	16	18	18	18	18	20	?	21	22	23	24	29	35
M.R.	12	F	23	20	18	17	17	16	17	17	17	17	18	20	22	23	23	26	31	32
N.M.S.	36	F	23	21	18	18	17	18	18	18	18	18	Rotated				27	30	33	
H.v.d.M.	14	F	22	20	18	18	18	17	18	18.5	18.5	19	20	22	23	24	26	26	?	?
E.T.	13	F	25	20	18	18	17	17	17.5	18	18.5	19.5	20.5	23	25	25	27	27	?	?
H.C.	30	F	22	19	18	17.5	18	17.5	17	17	17	18	18	20	?	22	22	25	27	?
J.C.	10	F	?	?	20	18	18	18.5	18.5	19	19	20	21	21.5	23.5	24	24	25	28	?
H.C.	4	M	25	20	18.5	17	18	18	18	18	18.5	18.5	21	22	22	22	22	22.5	23	?
L.C.	17	F	22	18	17	17	16.5	16	16	16.5	17	18	19	24	24	24	23	23	25	24

(mm)

The width of the inter-penduncular spaces of the thoracic and lumbar regions of the spine, as determined radiographically in 50 healthy individuals of all age groups and of both sexes. A number of cases of sub-clinical scoliosis is included in the series.

The narrow zone of the spinal canal which is indicated by a heavy horizontal line above, extends from T4 to T8 level in the majority of cases, and includes the 6th thoracic vertebra in 49 out of 50 individuals.

TABLE 8.2

**MEASUREMENTS OF THE LUMEN OF THE SPINAL CANAL
ANTERO-POSTERIOR & LATERAL DIMENSION (MILLIMETERS)
DEyARTMENT OF ANATOMY, UNIVERSITY OF PRETORIA**

VERT. LEVEL	CADAVER NUMBER											
	2806		2833		2751		2917A		2985		2917B	
	LAT	A-P	LAT	A-P	LAT	A-P	LAT	A-P	LAT	A-P	LAT	A-P
T1	22.7	13.8	21.3	14.4	22.3	15.0	17.8	13.7	21.7	15.9	18.2	12.8
T2	20.6	14.6	18.2	13.7	18.8	14.6	15.4	13.6	19.4	15.0	16.5	12.6
T3	18.7	14.6	16.5	13.6	16.5	16.3	14.4	13.5	17.7	15.1	15.7	12.8
T4	17.7	14.6	14.2	13.3	15.9	15.2	14.3	12.5	16.0	14.7	15.0	13.4
T5	17.7	14.2	14.6	12.9	15.1	14.1	14.0	12.0	15.4	14.5	14.1	13.9
T6	17.0	13.9	14.1	13.2	14.3	14.2	14.2	11.2	15.1	14.0	14.7	13.8
T7	16.7	14.1	15.3	12.2	14.2	14.2	13.9	12.2	15.3	14.4	15.2	14.2
T8	16.1	13.6	14.4	13.2	14.9	14.2	15.5	12.7	16.1	14.3	15.2	13.4
T9	16.6	13.9	15.2	12.3	15.0	14.5	15.0	13.1	16.8	14.5	14.7	15.4
T10	17.0	13.1	15.0	11.8	15.0	14.4	17.0	13.2	17.3	14.8	15.7	13.6
T11	17.3	13.6	15.4	12.0	15.3	14.8	18.3	15.0	17.1	14.9	16.0	14.3
T12	19.1	16.2	14.8	13.7	18.4	16.9	20.6	16.6	19.0	16.4	18.8	14.0
L1	21.1	15.7	16.8	14.0	21.0	17.0	20.0	15.6	22.2	16.3	21.3	13.6
L2	20.7	14.7	17.8	13.8	21.7	15.0	21.1	14.7	16.7	17.2	22.5	14.0
L3	22.0	14.7	17.9	12.7	21.7	15.0	21.0	13.9	17.7	16.0	22.3	14.9
L4	25.0	17.0	19.5	11.6	23.2	16.5	22.1	14.2	18.3	16.0	23.0	15.3
L5	28.4	18.0	22.4	10.6	24.4	18.0	24.0	13.7	19.1	14.7	26.0	17.9
L6			23.4	11.5								
S1	35.0	14.2	23.4	11.8	30.2	10.0	22.8	8.3	27.1	12.2	31.0	14.0

Ther narrowest zone of the spinal canal, in both the antero-posterior and lateral diameters is circumscribed by a thick line.

Unit of length: mm

80

9. The Venous Drainage of the Spinal Cord

The veins of the spinal cord at birth and the veins at adult stage resemble each other in all respects except size, and in the former they are relatively larger than at any other stage of post-natal development.

The study of the veins is more difficult than the arteries, because of the technical problem of achieving adequate filling, and on account of the close relationship of the veins of the cord and the plexiform network of Batson (Batson, 1940, 1942). A distinction between the two sets of veins is necessary for an understanding of either, and to this end, a diagrammatic representation which offers a panoramic view of the veins of the spine, the spinal cord and related structures is presented (Fig. 9.1).

Fig. 9.1   Diagrammatic representation of the veins of the spine and spinal cord.

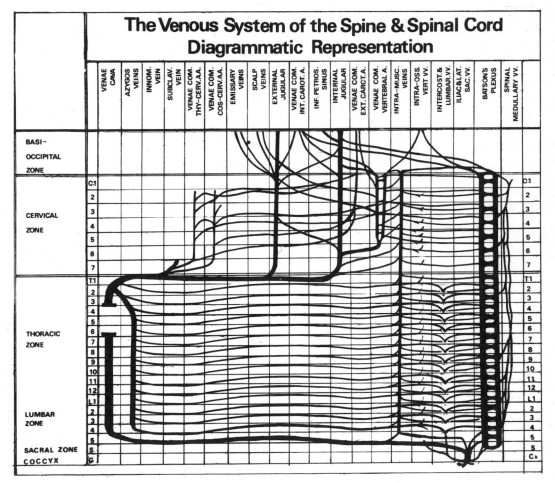

Spinal cord veins constitute a small yet vital component of the whole, and are represented here by a single, relatively insignificant column at the right extremity of the diagram. The relationship which the veins of the cord bear to those of the head, neck and trunk is important, as well as the fact of their drainage into the plexus of Batson, which is represented diagrammatically by a large, prominent column.

The extent of Batson's plexus is apparent, for it is not only the largest and most complex venous channel, but it is also the only venous system which extends from basi-occiput to coccyx, which communicates directly with both the superior and the inferior vena caval systems and at appropriate levels with the azygos system, and which forms an integral part of the venous drainage of both the brain and the spinal cord.

Spinal cord veins and the veins of Batson's plexus will be considered under separate subheadings. The terminology to be used has been outlined (see Chapter 2), and for easy reference is repeated.

TERMINOLOGY

1. The longitudinal venous trunks of the cord (Fig. 9.2). These are the anterior and posterior venous channels (Plates 20–24), which are the counterparts of the arterial trunks. Anteriorly there is a single trunk, which is placed over the anterior median sulcus deep to the arterial trunk (Plates 20, 21), and into it drain the central perforating and the pial perforating veins, also numerous radicular venules at every segment. At the cervical and lumbar enlargements it is often seen as a complex system of venous channels, which are abundant and may resemble arterio-venous malformations. Posteriorly a single midline trunk may be replaced in whole or in part by duplicated or ramifying vessels which are likewise abundant at the cervical and the lumbar enlargements of the cord (Plates 22–24). The longitudinal venous trunks of the cord drain into the inner, central portion of the plexus of Batson, that portion described below under the sub-title *the extra-dural vertebral venous plexus*.

2. The medullary veins of the cord (Plates 20–24). These are the counterparts of the medullary feeder arteries. They accompany the nerve roots in their

**THE ANTERIOR AND POSTERIOR LONGITUDINAL VENOUS CHANNELS OF THE SPINAL CORD
IN TWO CADAVERS, ONE INFANTILE & ONE ADULT.**

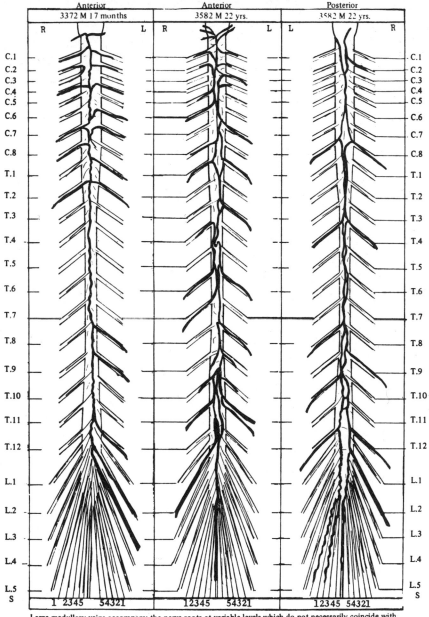

Large medullary veins accompany the nerve roots at variable levels which do not necessarily coincide with
the levels of the feeder arteries.
Radicular venules for the drainage of the nerve roots are present at all levels.

Fig. 9.2   The anterior and posterior longitudinal venous trunks of the spinal cord.

exit from the dural sac, at levels which are usually not related to the medullary feeder arteries.

They are largest and most constant at the cervical and the lumbar enlargements.

3. The extra-dural vertebral venous plexus (Plates 25–27). That portion of the plexus of Batson which occupies the extra-dural space of the spinal canal and extends from basi-occiput to coccyx.

It is illustrated here in the cervical, thoracic and lumbar regions.

There are other elements of Batson's plexus, which are described below, under *The venous plexus of Batson.*

4. The vertebral venous plexus (Plates 25, 28).

This term is used in the literature to denote the several components of the plexus of Batson and has become a sort of generic term, lacking definition.

In this presentation it is used in a specific sense, to denote the plexus of veins which surrounds the vertebral artery within the transverse foramen, and which communicates with the cervical portion of the extra-dural plexus at every segmental level. It communicates also with the veins of the neck, both deep and superficial. Proximally, it participates in the great confluence of venous sinuses (see below), which has hitherto not been fully described.

5. The great confluence of venous sinuses (Plate 25).

A complex, complicated venous network situated at the basi-occiput. Trevor-Jones (1966) refers to the multilateral communications in this area: 'The venous connection between the vertebral venous plexus and the internal jugular vein and inferior petrosal sinus have not been described before. Tobias and Arnold (1963) have drawn attention to the analogous nature of anastomoses between extracranial and intracranial and between extra- and intravertebral venous systems. The presence of these two connections on the superior aspect of the atlas completes the series.'

The participants in the great confluence of venous sinuses include:

A. Those emerging from the cranial cavity. They are

    i) The internal jugular veins (Plates 25, 28).

    ii) The inferior petrosal sinus (Plate 25).

    iii) Veins which accompany the internal carotid

artery, and multiple small veins which
emerge from the cranial cavity through
numerous foramina, named and unnamed.
iv) Emissary veins of the skull which empty into
scalp veins (Fig. 9.3).

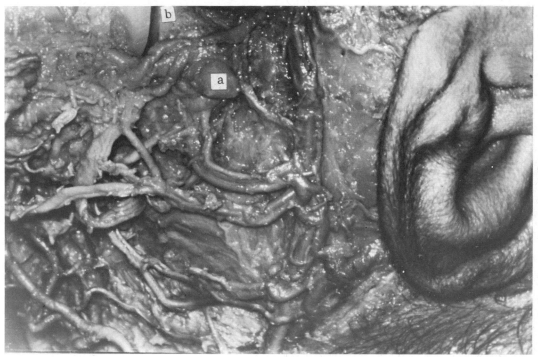

Fig. 9.3 The veins of the scalp draining distally and communicating directly with the deep veins of the neck and the great confluence of venous sinuses at basi-occiput. (a) Transverse process of C1 vertebra. (b) Paravertebral joint at C1/C2 level. Note the pinna of the ear is rotated upwards and the neck of the cadaver is extended through an angle of ninety degrees.

B. The deep veins of the neck, which include:
  i) The extradural, vertebral venous plexus
    (Plate 25).
  ii) The vertebral venous plexus (Plates 25, 28).
 iii) The veins which accompany the branches of
    the deep cervical and the ascending cervical
    arteries.
 iv) The veins of the anterior and posterior
    cervical muscles.
C. The superficial veins of the head and neck.
  i) The veins of the scalp (Fig. 9.3; Plate 28).
  ii) The veins which accompany the superficial
    branches of the external carotid artery
    (Plate 28).
D. The veins of the skull and the vertebral skeleton.

   i) A venous plexus within the clivus, with
        channels emerging from numerous small
        foramina (Plate 25).
  ii) A venous plexus within the bone trabeculae
        of the arch of the atlas, with channels
        emerging from the bony structure.
   Undoubtedly there are many other vessels which
participate in the great confluence. Trevor Jones (1966)
refers to a posterior group of veins at the occiput, thus:
'Postero-laterally, communications may be found
through the foramen magnum with the occipital sinus'.
The same writer adds: 'A large venous channel passes
superiorly and laterally across the lateral mass of the
atlas to join the internal jugular vein'. This channel is
illustrated below (Plates 25, 28).

Fig. 9.4 The posterior longitudinal
venous channels of the spinal cord
at from T11 to L1 vertebral levels.
The veins in this photograph are
filled with blood and are dark in
colour. The arterial channel on the
left side has been exposed by the
division of the posterior nerve
rootlets, and is shown to be tortuous
and 'rambling' in its course.

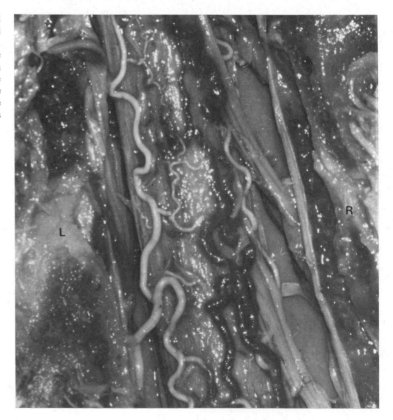

THE VEINS OF THE SPINAL CORD (Figs. 2.1, 9.4; Plates 20–24)

The veins of the cord resemble the arteries, and take the
form of pial perforating veins, longitudinal venous

trunks both anterior and posterior, and veins which are the counterpart of the medullary feeder arteries (Plates 21, 24). Radicular veins are for the drainage of the nerve roots as opposed to the medulla.

Suh and Alexander (1939) declared: 'The anterior radicular veins. essentially resemble in distribution the anterior radicular arteries', and they composed a set of diagrams in which they depicted the ventral and dorsal veins (also the ventral and dorsal arteries), of the spinal medulla. Their findings were in essential agreement with those of Kadyi (1889), and in turn have been corroborated in the present series.

Abrams (1957) recognised the direction of spinal cord drainage: 'Foreign substances in the spinal theca drain directly through the vertebral veins into the azygos system', and it is clear that the term 'vertebral veins' was used by Abrams in respect of the extradural portion of Batson's plexus.

A degree of confusion has however arisen, due to the fact that Batson's plexus was regarded as an extension of the veins of the cord, rather than as a venous channel into which the veins of the cord emptied, and one which subserved numerous other functions.

Suh and Alexander (1939) were impressed with the abundance of the venous channels: 'The observation which we . . . wish to emphasize is the striking difference in size between the various radicular arteries and veins in the spinal cord'. This remark cannot be supported in the present series, in which the veins were dissected out with the aid of the surgical microscope, and with the spinal cord *in situ*. It was found that the veins were commensurate with the arteries and that the product of the number and the sizes of the veins was approximately equal to that of the arteries, as long as the extradural veins were excluded from the reckoning.

Herlihy (1947) was under the same impression as Suh and Alexander and declared: '. . . that the venous system is much greater in volume than the arterial system, for often two veins occur with each artery, veins occur in regions where there are no arteries, and veins on the whole are larger than arteries'. The implication in each case was that venous outflow is greater than arterial inflow, and in each case, the explanation was probably based on venous reflux.

While the present observations support the theory of reflux in the plexiform network of Batson, they oppose the view of reflux in the veins of the spinal medulla, for two reasons. First, the medullary veins are in fact no more abundant than the arteries, and second, the axillary pouches of the dural sac, at which the veins make their exit in the company of the segmental nerve roots, appear to serve the function of venous valves. Retrograde filling of the medullary veins was successful in relatively few cadavers in this series.

There is a third factor, which was expressed by Stephens and Stillwell (1969), in respect of the brain and which can probably be applied also to the spinal cord. The metabolic activity of neural tissue is high, and the consumption of oxygen is about ten times greater than elsewhere, in the basal state. The circulating blood volume is proportional to the demand, and there is no room for the storage of venous blood either in the brain or in the spinal cord. The theory of venous reflux would appear totally unacceptable, in the cord just as in the brain, and the importance of drawing a distinction between the veins of the cord on the one hand, and of Batson's plexus on the other, would appear to be re-emphasised.

Fig. 9.5 The extra-vertebral venous plexus in the neck, on the surface of the longus colli muscle. It communicates laterally with the segmental veins of the cervical vertebrae.

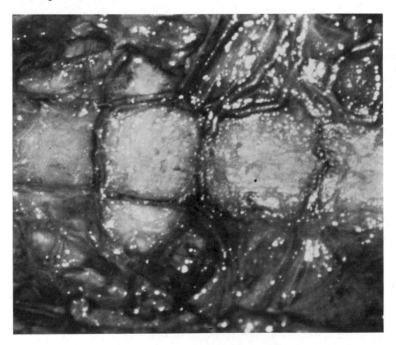

THE VENOUS PLEXUS OF BATSON (Fig. 9.1)
The magnitude of the great plexiform network of veins

which extends throughout the length of the vertebral column, from basi-occiput to sacrum was first described by Breschet (1832), whose contribution is acknowledged by Batson (1940). He demonstrated the relationship between the veins of the skull and the vertebral column.

Batson demonstrated the spread of metastatic emboli from the pelvis to the brain via the vertebral portion of the network which he termed 'the vertebral veins' and added 'they have connections with the veins in the spinal canal, . . . around the spinal column, . . . and within the bones of the column'. He injected the dorsal vein of the penis in an adult cadaver with a thin radiopaque material which could be made to by-pass the inferior vena cava and to reach the base of the skull and the cranial cavity through the medium of 'the veins about the dura and those in and about the vertebrae'. He commented: 'Although the vertebral plexus of veins . . . was familiar ground from our earlier preparations, we were not prepared for this extensive filling of the vertebral veins and the by-passing of the caval veins. . . . (It) furnished a composite picture of the metastatic pattern of . . . carcinomatosis . . . in the prostate.' Batson proceeded to duplicate the experiment in the living animal, and succeeded with the Macassus Rhesus monkey when he tied a towel about the animal's abdomen in order to obstruct the inferior vena cava. He concluded that the vena cava offered the normal drainage under conditions of trunk muscle inactivity, but that the 'vertebral system of veins' was responsible for some of the drainage under conditions of increased intra-abdominal pressure such as produced in coughing or straining (Batson, 1940).

The three component parts of Batson's plexus are:

1. The extra-dural, vertebral venous plexus described above (Plates 25–27).
2. The extra-vertebral venous plexus which includes the segmental veins of the neck (Fig. 9.5), the intercostal veins and the azygos communications in the thorax (Fig. 9.6), the lumbar veins and the azygos communications in the pelvis, and the communications with the inferior vena caval system (Fig. 9.7).
3. The veins of the bony structures of the spinal column. They are described elsewhere, Crock *et al.* (1973). They communicate freely with 1 and 2 above by means of thin-walled channels which

emerge from the nutrient foramina of the vertebrae within and without the spinal canal respectively.

Herlihy (1947), whose untimely death 20 years ago in Australia undoubtedly prevented a flow of scholarly contributions, defined the functions of the 'vertebral venous plexus' in terms of the 'anatomy of the veins themselves, and it will be found that the description fits in well with what we have now formulated in our mind.

(*a*) It is a storehouse of blood, and this we see in the architecture of its dilations and in its very magnitude.

(*b*) It is a pool for receiving backflow from adjacent veins, hence its many anastomoses.

(*c*) It redistributes the blood from other adjacent parts, and the backflow from other regions is soon accommodated in its very immensity. It reminds us of the invaders of China, who are absorbed until they themselves become Chinese.

(*d*) Any unequal pressure in adjacent veins is quickly equalized, and this follows as a result of the greatness of the system's extent, its low pressure . . . and the dilatations in each segment.

(*e*) It itself has no pressure, and hence is more suitable to act as a pressure absorber.

(*f*) It has no direction of flow, and this makes possible a quick adjustment and accommodation to a sudden inrush of blood; this is shown in its consisting of a network instead of longitudinal channels'.

Herlihy's writings possess a charm and forthrightness which are a delight to the reader and at the same time a source of sorrow at the early passing of a great observer. It is perhaps not strange, and it is worth recording that beneath the title of the contribution recorded here, he wrote what might have been his own epitaph: 'The simple believeth every word; but the prudent man looketh well to his going'—Proverbs XIV, 15.

Batson (1940) commented on the structure of veins: 'The strictly vertebral portion of the network is composed of thin-walled vessels; when empty of blood they are difficult to identify yet they have considerable volume'.

In the present series, they have repeatedly impressed the observer with the thinness of their walls and with the unpredictability of their successful filling. They are present in all age groups but are overlooked when not filled with the injection material. When successfully filled, they are massive and form a delicate tracery which

continued on p. 92

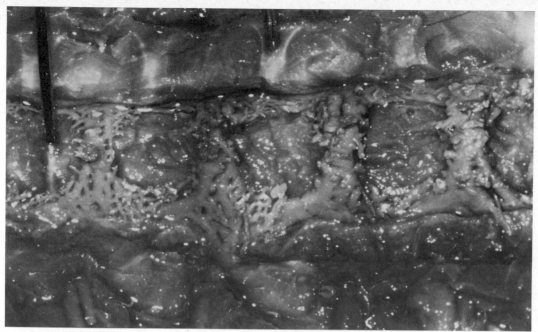

Fig. 9.6   The communications between the extradural plexus, and the extravertebral veins, namely the intercostal and azygos veins.

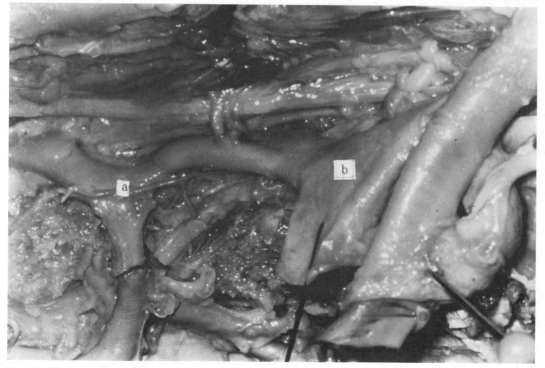

Fig. 9.7   The extra-dural venous plexus (a), communicating with the left internal iliac vein (b), here shown divided.

cannot be handled without damage, even with the finest
forceps. They may be displayed by a careful dissection
and removal of the surrounding tissues, with the aid of a
surgical microscope.

Batson demonstrated the passage of injection material
from the pelvis and the breast to the brain along the
venous channels of the vertebral column. The direction
of the flow of blood and the potential for the blood-
bourne spread of metastatic emboli by way of the
venous plexus were established.

In the present study, it was postulated and later
demonstrated that a flow of blood in the reverse
direction, that is, in a distal direction, could also take
place. The reversibility of the direction of flow which
was described by Batson, is important to the thesis put
forward here, namely that the veins of the spinal cord
drain into the extra-dural vertebral venous plexus.

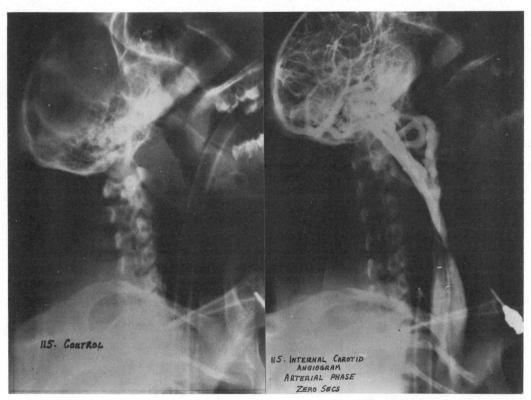

Fig. 9.8a, b   Carotid angiogram using an experimental animal, the baboon *Papio ursinus*. a. The cannula in position
in the internal carotid artery. b. On completion of the injection of 20 cc., Urografin 76 per cent. The arterial phase.
Note rapid and immediate venous filling. c. Venous phase, at 6 seconds after completion of injection of contrast
medium, under normal conditions. d. Venous phase, at 6 seconds, after ligation of both internal jugular veins. The
external jugular veins with a little assistance from Batson's plexus are immediately effective.

Animal experimentation, using six baboons of the species *Papio ursinus* were carried out as follows:

The animals were anaesthetised and an intra-tracheal tube was inserted.

A carotid angiogram was carried out by means of a cannula inserted in the carotid artery, by an open dissection. The blind introduction of a large cannula was difficult and gave rise to haematoma formation.

The injection of 20 ml of a 76 per cent solution of Urogafin was followed by a series of radiographic films, taken at intervals of one second, in which both the arterial and the venous phases were observed.

The normal venous drainage of the brain was seen to take place through the internal jugular veins (Fig. 9.8B, C). In some specimens a minor spill-over into the plexus of Batson was observed. When the internal jugular veins on both sides were ligated, then drainage took place through the external jugular veins (Fig. 9.8). When both the internal and both the external jugulars were ligated, then drainage took place through the

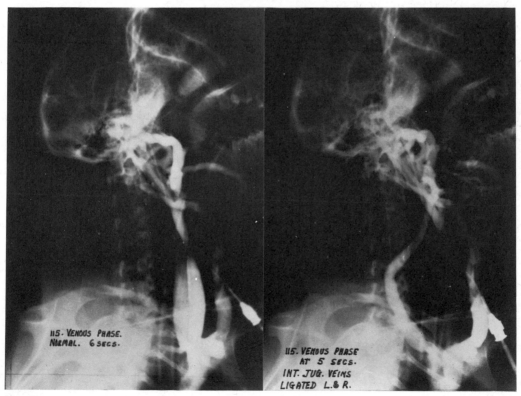

Fig. 9.8c   Fig. 9.8d

extra-dural vertebral portion of Batson's plexus (Fig. 9.8e). Under radiological television screening, the rapid, unhesitating diversion of the venous blood to Batson's plexus was impressive, and the speed with which the venous phase was reached and completed was unaffected.

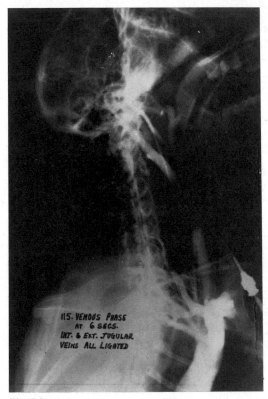

Fig. 9.8e

e. Venous phase, at 6 seconds, after ligation of both internal and both external jugular veins. The plexus of Batson is rapidly effective in accomplishing the venous drainage of the brain and constitutes an efficient alternative pathway.

There were no obvious adverse effects on the animals, and the procedure was repeated in two animals eighteen days later. The results were the same.

These animal experiments, when taken in conjunction with those of Batson (1940, 1942), serve to confirm the potential for a flow of blood in either direction, and to draw attention to earlier comments on the Harveian concept of the circulation.

Herlihy commented to the effect that although the circulation is from heart to arteries and back to the heart through the veins, the truth is, in fact, 'something much less simple'. He declared: 'I wish to draw special attention to the pool of blood in the vertebral veins. The functions of this plexus—equilibrization of pressure, reception of back flow and redistribution with respiration et cetera—have been mentioned. In and out of this plexus blood runs, not unlike the earliest conceptions of an "ebb and flow". . . . Eventually all the blood returns to the heart, but not in a continuous circle as Harvey would have. The realization of this is of the utmost importance in anatomy, physiology, pathology and surgery'.

The anatomical configuration of the venous channels of Batson as displayed in the current series, support the contentions of both Herlihy and Batson who commented: 'According to the concept here developed we have a vast system of veins which on the ground of anatomic injections, animal experiments, and simple logic, is constantly and physiologically the site of frequent reversals of flow. During these reversals a pathway exists up and down the spine which does not involve the heart or the lungs'. (Note: The comments of the above two authors are not applicable to spinal cord veins, but only to the plexiform network which is Batson's plexus.)

Herbert Abrams (1957) has added to the knowledge of the plexus of Batson, which remains a field for further fruitful research.

In the current series, the distinction between the veins of the spinal cord on the one hand and the plexiform venous network of Batson on the other, appears important, more particularly in view of the fact that the metabolic requirements of the neural tissues of the cord are far in excess of those of other tissues, that the arterial supply of the cord is 'only just adequate for its needs' (Feeney and Watterson, 1946), and that the venous channels of the cord are commensurate with the arterial vessels. The alternative routes of venous drainage which are offered by this ubiquitous network of venous channels, are an apparent safeguard or 'safety valve' in the event of focal venous obstruction. The theory of a safety valve proffered here is attractive, and provides a venous counterpart for the arterial 'safety valve' which has been demonstrated in this series in the form of arterial circles, also by Woollam and Millen (1958) who liken the arterial anastomoses to the circle of Willis, and by Lazorthes *et al.* (1971), who describe 'substitution arterial pathways'.

The theory is doubly attractive, for it helps to bridge the gap between the physiological fact of the spinal cord which has 'a blood supply just adequate for its minimal needs' (Feeney and Watterson, 1946), and the clinical fact of cord 'immunity' or cord escape, in the presence of major injury involving segmental vertebral arteries as well as the ramifications of Batson's plexus.

The subject offers an attractive field for investigation, in which may be included the pathogenesis of such widely divergent entities as degenerative myelopathy and idiopathic scoliosis.

10. The Segmental Arteries of Supply

Segmental arteries are present on both sides of the spinal column at every level and they are as vital to cord supply as the internal carotid and the vertebral arteries are to the brain (Principle 1, p. 17).

They supply a number of structures other than the cord and together constitute an integrated system of supply which is linked by means of arterio-arterial anastomoses (circles), across the middle line, and between ipsi-lateral neighbours (Plates 18, 19).

The nerve roots at every level and on both sides of the midline are supplied by radicular vessels (Plates 11, 27).

Other structures include:

1. **The sympathetic ganglia** (Fig. 10.1) which derive their supply from regional branches of the segmental vessels. There is a considerable variability in the source, but in all instances the ganglionic supply is abundant.

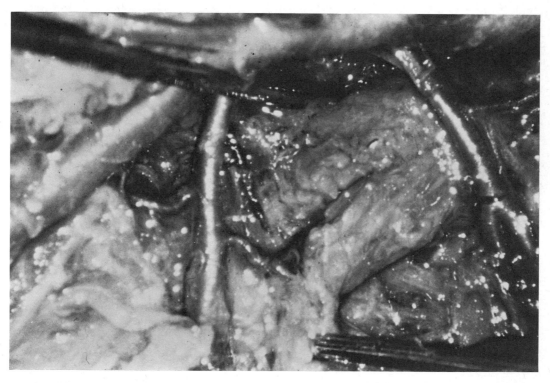

Fig. 10.1   The inferior cervical ganglion on the left side. In this instance the blood supply is from the superior intercostal artery. The ganglia enjoy a rich supply.

2. **The autonomic nerve trunks.** The sympathetic trunks are abundantly supplied (Plate 29), like the segmental nerve roots.
3. **The paravertebral muscles** (Fig. 10.2). The muscles are richly supplied, but the supply is unilateral and there is minimum crossing of the midline by muscular branches. This fact has been noted by Harrington (1969) and others, and is of practical significance and value in posterior surgical approaches.

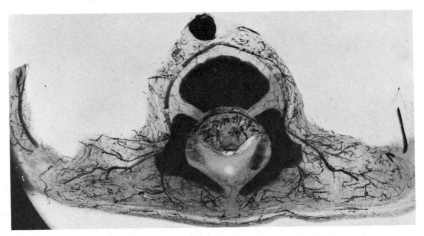

Fig. 10.2   Cross-section of the paravertebral muscles at lumbar level. The arteries of supply are from the aortic segmental vessels, and they follow the course of the primary rami of the posterior divisions of the nerve roots.

4. **The vertebral skeleton** is supplied by nutrient vessels which enter the bodies along the course of the segmental arteries towards the intervertebral foramina (Plate 9). These arteries are distinguished by their numbers rather than their calibre. Major nutrient arteries enter the vertebral bodies via nutrient foramina situated at the posterior aspect, and via branches of a transverse, extra-dural arterial circle (Plate 17), which perforate the posterior longitudinal ligament at several places. A large vascular 'nubbin' is seen at the midpoint of the posterior surface of the vertebral body, through which nutrient arteries make their entrance and veins gain exit. The posterior, neural arches are supplied by vessels which branch off from the parent segmental artery at the intervertebral foramen. They were described by Macnab and Dall (1971).

THE MEMBRANES OF THE SPINAL CANAL
Surrounding the dura mater, and incorporating the
posterior longitudinal ligament of the spine, is a thick,
double-layered membrane (Plate 30) which at the
posterior portion of the spinal canal incorporates the thin
periosteal lining of the neural arch. Between its layers
are some of the veins of the extradural portion of
Batsons' plexus, while between it and the dura mater are
the transverse segmental venous channels. The membrane
is one of great dimension and is not generally recognised
as a separate entity. It is generally mistaken for the
'outer layer of the dura'. It requires further study in
conditions of health and of disease.

In conclusion, an appreciation of the close
relationship between the vessels of the spinal cord, the
bony skeleton, the spinal musculature, the nerve roots
and the autonomic nerve trunks and ganglia is
fundamental to the study of spinal cord circulation, and
to a breakdown into its component parts, of the
somewhat overwhelming global system of arterial supply
and venous drainage.

REFERENCES

ABRAMS, H. L. (1957) The vertebral and azygos venous systems, and some variations in systemic venous return. *Radiology,* **69,** 508.

ADAMKIEWICZ, A. A. (1881a) Ueber die mikroskopischen Gefässe des menschlichen Rückenmarkes. *Trans. 7th Session, Int. Med. Congress,* **1,** 155–157.

ADAMKIEWICZ, A. A. (1881b) Die Blutgefässe des Menslichen Ruckemarkes; 1. Die Gefässe der Ruckenmarkssubstanz. Situngsb.d.k. Akad. d. Wissensch., Math.-naturw. Cl. 84: 469.

ADAMKIEWICZ, A. A. (1882) Die Blutgefässe des menschlichen Rückenmarkes: II. Die Gefässe der Rückenmarksoberfläche, Situngsb.d.k. Akad. d. Wissensch., Math.-naturw. Cl. 85: 101–130.

ALEXANDER, L. & PUTNAM, T. J. (1938) Pathological alterations of cerebral vascular patterns. *Arch. Research Nerv. & Ment. Dis., Proc.,* **18,** 471.

BATSON, O. V. (1940) The function of the vertebral veins and their rôle in the spread of metastases. *Ann. Surg.,* **112,** 138.

BATSON, O. V. (1942) The vertebral vein system as a mechanism for the spread of metastases. *Am. J. Roentgenol. Rad. Therapy,* **48,** 6, 715.

BOLTON, B. (1939) The blood supply of the human spinal cord. *J. Neurol. Psychiat.,* **1–2,** 137.

BRESCHET, G. (1832) *Recherches Anatomiques, Physiologiques et Pathologiques sur le systéme vieneux.* Paris.

CHAKRAVORTY, B. G. (1969) The arterial supply of the cervical cord and its relation to cervical spondylosis in myelopathy. *Ann. Roy. Col. Surg. Eng.,* **45,** 232.

CROCK, H. V., YOSHIZAWA, H. & KAME, S. K. (1973) Observations on the venous drainage of the human vertebral body. *J. Bone and Joint Surg.,* **55,** 528.

DICHIRO, G., FRIED, L. C. and DOPPMAN, J. L. (1970) Experimental spinal cord angiography. *Br. J. Radiol.,* **43,** 19.

DJINDJIAN, R. with HURST, M. *et al.* (1970) *Angiography of the spinal cord.* L'Angiographic de la Moelle épinére. Masson & Kie, Paries. Univ. Baltimore: Park Press.

DOMMISSE, G. F. (1972a) The blood supply of the human spinal cord at birth. Ch.M. Thesis, University of Cape Town.

DOMMISSE, G. F. (1972b) Some factors in the management of fractures and fracture-dislocations of the spine at lumbo-dorsal level. The significance of the blood supply. *Recon. Surg. & Traumatol.,* **13,** 108.

DOMMISSE, G. F. (1974a) The blood supply of the spinal cord. A critical vascular zone in spinal surgery. *J. Bone and Joint Surg.,* British Volume, 56B: 225.

DOMMISSE, G. F. (1974b) Vascular system of the human spinal cord. M.D. Thesis, University of Pretoria.

DWYER, A. F. (1972) Personal communication.

FEENEY, J. F. & WATTERSON, R. L. (1946) The development of the vascular pattern within the walls of the central nervous system of the chick embryo. *J. Morphol.,* **78,** 231.

FRIED, L. C., DOPPMAN, J. L. & DICHIRO, G. (1970) Direction of blood flow in the primate cervical spinal cord. *J. Neurosurg.,* **33,** 325.

HALL, J. E. (1973) Personal communication.

HARRINGTON, P. R. (1969) Personal communication.

HARRIS, R. (1973) Traction lesions of the lumbo-sacral plexus in fractures of the pelvis with sacro-iliac subluxation. Paper read at Annual meeting of *Am. Orth. Assn., June 1970,* and quoted by F. P. Dewar (1973) in a personal communication.

HARVEY, W. (1628) Exercitatio de motu cordis et sanguinis in animalibus. Francofurti, G. Fitzeri. (Translations R. Willis (1889) and H. J. Franklin (1957).

HERLIHY, W. F. (1947) Revision of the venous system: The rôle of the vertebral veins. *Med. J. Australia,* **22,** 661.

KADYI, H. (1889) Ueber die Blutgefässe des menschliche Rückenmarkes; nach einer im XV. Bande der Denkschriften der mach.-naturw. Classe der Akademie der Wissenschaften in Krakau erschienenen Monographie, aus dem Polnischen übersetzt vom Verfasser, Lemberg, Poland, Gubrynowicz & Schmidt.

KEIM, H. A. & HILAL, S. K. (1971) Spinal angiography in scoliosis patients. *J. Bone and Joint Surg.,* **53A,** 904.

LAZORTHES, G., GOUAZE, A., ZADEH, J. O., SANTINI, J. J., LAZORTHES, Y. and BURDIN, P. (1971) Arterial vascularization of the spinal cord. Recent studies of the anastomotic substitution pathways. *J. Neurosurg.,* **35,** 253.

MACNAB, I. and DALL, D. (1971) The blood supply of

the lumbar spine and its application to the technique of intertransverse lumbar fusion. *J. Bone and Joint Surg.*, **53B**, 628.

PATTEN, B. M. (1968b) *Human Embryology*. 3rd Edition. McGraw-Hill Book Company. The Blakiston Div. New York, Toronto, Sydney, London.

ROMANES, G. J. (1965) The arterial blood supply of the human spinal cord. *Paraplegia.*, **2**, 299.

ROSSOUW, A. (1972) Personal communication.

SCHLEGEL, J. E. (1945) Arteriovenous anastomoses in the endometrium in man. *Acta Anat.*, **1**, 284.

STEPHENS, R. B. and STILLWELL, D. L. (1969) *Arteries and veins of the human brain*. Springfield, Illinois: Charles C. Thomas.

STREETER, G. I. (1918) The developmental alterations in the vascular system of the brain of the human embryo. In *Contributions to Embryology,* pp. 7–38. Washington: Carnegie Institute.

SUH, T. H. and ALEXANDER, L. (1939) Vascular system of the human spinal cord. *Arch. Neurol. Psychiat.*, **41**, 659.

TOBIAS, P. V. and ARNOLD, M. (1963) *Man's Anatomy*. Vol. II. p. 265. Johannesburg: Witwatersrand University Press.

TREVOR-JONES, R. (1966) Vascular changes occurring in the cervical muscle-skeletal system. *S.A. Med. J.*, **40**, 388.

TRUETA, J., BARCLAY, A. E., DANIEL, P. M., FRANKLIN, K. J. and PRICHARD, M. M. L. (1947) *Studies of the Renal Circulation*. Oxford: Blackwell.

TURNBULL, I. M. (1971) Microvasculature of the human spinal cord. *J. Neurosurg.*, **35**, 141.

WISSDORF, H. (1970) Die Gefässversorgung der Wirbel Säule und des Rückenmarkes vom Hausschewein (SVS Scrofa Domestica L., 1758). *Beiheft iz zum zentralblatt für Veterinärmedizin*. Berlin en Hamburg: Verlag, Paul Parey.

WOLMAN, L. (1965) The disturbance of circulation in traumatic paraplegia in acute and late stages: A pathological study. *Paraplegia,* **2,** 213.

WOOLLAM, D. H. M. and MILLEN, J. W. (1958) In Discussion on vascular diseases of the spinal cord. *Proc. Roy. Soc. Med.*, **51**, 540.

YORKE HERREN, R. and LEO ALEXANDER (1939) Sulcal and intrinsic blood vessels of human spinal cord. *Arch. Neurol. Psychiat.*, **41**, 678,

Index

Printed by T. & A. Constable Ltd.,
Hopetoun Street,
EDINBURGH

Filmset by Typesetting Services Ltd.,
Glasgow and Edinburgh